Surrogates & Other Mothers

The Debates Over Assisted Reproduction

RUTH MACKLIN

Surrogates

& Other Mothers

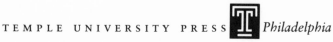

TEMPLE UNIVERSITY PRESS **T** *Philadelphia*

Temple University Press,
Philadelphia 19122
Copyright © 1994 by Ruth Macklin
All rights reserved
Published 1994
Printed in the United States
of America

Library of Congress
Cataloging-in-Publication Data

Macklin, Ruth, 1938–

Surrogates and other mothers : the
debates over assisted reproduction /
Ruth Macklin.

p.   cm.

Includes bibliographical references
and index.

ISBN 1-56639-179-2.—ISBN
1-56639-180-6 (pbk.)

1. Human reproductive
technology—Moral and ethical
aspects. 2. Surrogate motherhood—
Moral and ethical aspects. 3. Pregnant
women—Legal status, laws, etc.
4. Fetus—Legal status, laws, etc.
I. Title.
RG133.5.M33   1994
176—dc20   93-5988

For my mother, of course

Contents

Acknowledgments

I am grateful to my colleagues at Albert Einstein College of Medicine, to the medical students, house staff, and other contributors to conferences that supplied much of the case material for this book. Thanks also go to members of the New Jersey Task Force on New Reproductive Practices and to the capable staff of the New Jersey Bioethics Commission. Informal presentations at meetings and documents prepared by staff were valuable resources, as was the final report of the task force, *After Baby M: The Legal, Ethical and Social Dimensions of Surrogacy.*

Some material is adapted or excerpted from my previously published work, as noted in the credits at the end of the book. I thank the editors and publishers of those works for permission to use the material.

Special thanks go to my friend Marie Burnett, for her thorough editorial work on the entire manuscript and for her insights and expertise in psychology. The encouragement and support of Jane Cullen at Temple University Press were great assets from beginning to end, and I am grateful to Patricia Sterling for her skillful editing of the final version of the manuscript.

My initial research and preliminary ideas for the book were formulated during a sabbatical semester several years ago under a grant award from the American Council of Learned Societies. I thank the ACLS for that support, which enabled me to launch this project.

Introduction

The world of modern medicine is constantly in flux. New problems sometimes arise out of nature; others result from scientific or technological advances; still others represent novel social arrangements. Together these problems challenge health professionals, lawyers, policymakers, and citizens to arrive at satisfactory solutions. This book depicts an array of unprecedented challenges to ethics, law, and public policy stemming from new developments in biomedicine.

A technological advance that has produced legal and ethical dilemmas is the expansion of medical techniques to combat infertility. A related development, the new reproductive practice known as "surrogacy," has confounded public policy. Progress in maternal-fetal medicine has given rise to a set of complications falling under the heading "maternal-fetal conflict." A biological novelty is the appearance of a new and deadly infectious disease: AIDS. These and other issues can become intertwined, creating legal and ethical quandaries both for professionals and for ordinary citizens whose lives are touched by these problems.

The topics addressed in this book are subjects about which people have profound and deeply rooted feelings. The pain and suffering that accompany infertility; the desperate longing for a genetically related, "perfect" baby; fear, anger, and feelings of vindictiveness surrounding the AIDS epidemic—these are only some of the emotional factors that complicate personal decision-making and rational policy formation.

The vehicle I have chosen for presenting and analyzing these issues is an extended hypothetical case, centering on an infertile couple and people with whom they come in contact (whose names, of course, are all fictitious). As the couple's tale unfolds, the ensuing personal, ethical, legal, and social problems are addressed by other characters representing the medical and legal professions, prominent religious and ideological positions, and other relevant points of view. This format enables me to present a large body of diverse information in a narrative style that helps to convey the emotional force of the subject matter. Meetings of a government-appointed task force and a hospital ethics committee are used to demonstrate both the deliberative process and the substantive content of the work of actual groups grappling with these issues in our society today.

The inspiration for this book grew out of an oral presentation I was invited to make at a regional meeting of the American Academy of Psychiatry and the Law in 1988. The conference topic, "The New Sexual Issues" in psychiatry and law, was divided into three sections: surrogacy, AIDS, and new diagnostic categories (including premenstrual syndrome, or PMS). My task was to talk about the ethical aspects of these disparate concerns. Struggling to incorporate all three in a coherent presentation, I hit upon the idea of using a single hypothetical case to illustrate an array of contemporary bioethical and legal issues. The narrative device was a mechanism for introducing the subject matter and keeping the audience awake.

Although my hypothetical case may seem forced, since it is unlikely that the various events and circumstances depicted could happen to any one couple, the episodes depicted are all based on real clinical cases and situations drawn from current medical, psychiatric, legal, and bioethical literature; on agendas taken up by hospital ethics committees; and on actual attempts of a task force or drafting committee to devise policy statements.

The ethical, legal, and policy dilemmas presented in the book derive from my own experiences as a professional bioethicist working in a large urban medical center. These include serving concurrently on three hospital ethics committees in New York City, as well as on an ethics advisory committee to a clinic that provides fertility services; participating in a regional study section on ethical, legal, and social issues related to AIDS; conducting a monthly seminar in forensic psychiatry for practicing forensic psychiatrists, fellows, and psychiatric residents; and engaging in various clinical activities in an academic medical center.

In addition, I served on the Task Force on New Reproductive Practices appointed in 1988 by the New Jersey Commission on Legal and Ethical Problems in the Delivery of Health Care and was charged with making recommendations on surrogacy. The report of the task force, *After Baby M: The Legal, Ethical and Social Dimensions of Surrogacy*, was published in September 1992. Portions of several chapters of this book are patterned after discussions and presentations at task force meetings.

My work involves grappling with dilemmas regarding patients with HIV infection; dealing with novel situations posed by infertile individuals or couples seeking assisted reproduction; and mediating disagreements between health professionals about the right course of action when patients defy hospital rules or refuse recommended medical treatments, or when pregnant women's actions are deemed to be against the best interests of the fetus or the child. In some instances statutes or court decisions provide a solution to these ethical quandaries, but the statutory solution can vary from state to state, and lower court decisions are often overturned by higher courts.

This book aims to bring these complex and varied contemporary concerns to the reader in a lively and interesting way. Rather than present controversial issues in the usual philosophical style of "on one hand, on the other hand," I have chosen to put opposing arguments in the mouths of health professionals, lawyers, members of the clergy, feminists, a bioethicist, and ordinary folks. Annotated material—often appearing in single quotation marks within dialogue—is quoted from sources identified in the notes. The words ascribed to the Catholic priest are taken from published materials and from discussion at task force meetings in which I participated. The feminist depicted in the book represents "radical" feminism, but "liberal" feminism is also described. The disputes over the treatment of HIV-infected patients reflect actual conversations among physicians, nurses, and social workers.

This diverse subject matter is tied together by the experiences, thoughts, and feelings of the infertile couple—"Bonnie" and "Larry"—and the people in their lives, and it is linked thematically by my perspective, which draws on the panoply of issues encountered in the day-to-day work of a hospital bioethicist and a participant in policy deliberations on state, national, and nongovernmental commissions. Here, then, is a glimpse of the up-to-date world of bioethics, employing ethical analysis, citing legal developments, and, where possible, providing resolutions to deeply felt dilemmas.

Confronting Infertility

The trip home is a two-hour drive. Larry and Bonnie, a couple in their mid-thirties, say goodbye to Larry's family after a festive Thanksgiving dinner.

"You want me to drive?" Bonnie asks Larry. "Are you sleepy?"

"No, I'm fine," Larry replies, settling himself behind the wheel. "Fun Thanksgiving, huh Bon?"

"Mmm-hmm."

"What's wrong? I hope you're not going to start complaining again about how my mother treats you."

"No, it's not that. She was Okay."

"Come on, Bonnie, something's the matter. Tell me."

"It's the same old thing. I always get depressed when we're around families with kids. What's wrong with us, Larry? We've been trying for almost two years now."

"It takes a lot of couples a long time. You know that. Just be patient."

"Look at your brother and sister-in-law. They had their first baby ten months to the day after they got married."

"I wish you wouldn't compare me with my brother."

"I'm not; I'm just saying lots of people have no trouble at all getting pregnant. I feel useless. I keep thinking there's something wrong with us. I bet everyone else thinks so, too."

"Bonnie, you're imagining things. No one is sitting around judging us. Plenty of people actually choose not to have kids."

"Well, not us. We always knew we wanted a family. Even before we got married."

"Are you saying it was a mistake for us to get married? That we're not meant for each other?"

"No, Larry. But at this point, it seems we're officially an infertile couple."

"What do you mean, 'officially'?"

"I've been doing some reading. The standard medical definition of infertility is 'the inability of a couple to conceive after twelve months of intercourse without contraception.'"[1] Bonnie takes a pamphlet out of her purse. "It says so right here."

"Say the definition again?"

"The inability of a couple to conceive after 12 months of intercourse without contraception."

"Why does it say 'couple'? Either the husband is infertile or the wife is, right?"

"Yes, but these days the emphasis is on the couple. That's so no one gets blamed, I guess. See, it says here: 'Fertility is the product of interaction between two people and so the infertile *patient* is in effect the infertile *couple*.'"[2]

"What if an infertile couple gets divorced? It's still one person or the other who's infertile."

"Larry, what are you quibbling about? This is *our* problem, not just mine or yours."

"Mine? How could it be mine?"

"Sometimes it's the man who has the problem, you know."

"Of course I know that. But I don't think it's me. There's no history of infertility in my family."

"What does that show? There's none in mine either," Bonnie says. "You know, there are doctors who specialize in problems of infertility. Maybe we should go see one."

"I don't like the idea."

"Why not?"

"They start poking and sticking needles into you, giving you drugs and doing all sorts of tests. I'm a healthy guy. I believe in going to doctors only when you're sick."

"Infertility *is* a disease," Bonnie asserts.

"That's ridiculous. We're not sick. We function perfectly. People who have a disease can't function. They can't go to work, can't make love, don't feel good. We don't have any of those problems. How can you call infertility a disease?"

"It's not my definition. It's what some of these experts are saying. If doctors can treat it, then it must be a disease. Besides, you're wrong about our being able to function. We can't function the way we want to. I want to be a mother. We want to be parents. I feel miserable whenever we're with friends who have children. My parents can't wait to have grandchildren. Let's face it, Larry, infertility is a disease and we've got it!"

"I think we should stop talking about what's wrong with us—or you or me—and start doing something. Going to a doctor may cure a disease, but there's another way to solve our problem. Why don't we just go ahead and adopt?"

"We've already gone round and round on that one, Larry."

"Well, I'm suggesting it again."

"It's so difficult."

"What's so difficult? You go to the adoption agency, put your name on a list, wait for your number to come up, and that's all there is to it."

"But wouldn't you rather have a child with our genes?" Bonnie asks.

"I don't think that much about genes. If my son can play basketball, what difference does it make whether he has my genes or not? Maybe he'd do better with some other guy's genes. How about a high school basketball star who knocks up the prom queen and she gives the baby up for adoption?"

"Larry, you're so crude. But maybe you're right. Maybe we should try adoption," Bonnie says. "It's not as easy as you make it sound, though. I was talking to a woman I work with who adopted. Jenny and her husband had to wait six years for a baby."

"Six years! We'll be over forty by then! That's too old to start raising kids."

"Jenny said it's hard to get a baby that doesn't have birth defects."

"How come?"

"It's sad, but some people who have babies born with handicaps decide not to raise them, so they give them up for adoption."

"I wouldn't want a handicapped baby either."

"No one does, Larry, but that doesn't mean you should just give it away. A baby isn't like a broken appliance."

"Well, at least when you adopt a baby you have a choice. I'm certainly opposed to adopting a handicapped baby. What about you?"

"I'm not so sure. We could give some poor baby a wonderful home."

"Bonnie, life is tough enough as it is. Let's just go for a normal kid, Okay? What do we have to do to start the ball rolling?"

"I'll call Jenny; she knows a lot about it. Maybe we won't have to go through an agency. I'll find out what I can. You could ask around, too, you know."

"I don't mind. This will give us something positive to do for a change."

Larry and Bonnie fall silent as they continue the drive home. They look forward to beginning the process of arranging to adopt a baby.

❁

Bonnie learns from her co-worker that in their state there are two primary ways for adoption to take place: private placement, and agency-arranged adoption. In a private arrangement a child is placed directly with the adoptive family. Agency adoptions are conducted either by private agencies licensed by the state, or by the state's own child welfare agency. The agency is responsible for placing the child with an adoptive family that it has investigated and approved.[3] Since Bonnie and Larry don't know anyone with whom they might arrange a private placement, they decide to go to a private agency. Bonnie telephones to gather information. She is put in touch with a social worker at the agency.

"Yes, how may I help you?" asks Lola Winston.

"My name is Bonnie Roberts. My husband and I are interested in adopting."

"You'll have to come into the agency in person for an initial interview. That's how we begin. We have to determine a family's appropriateness for adoption. Following the initial interview, a home study process begins. The whole thing takes several months to complete."

"Several months? Is there a long wait for a baby?"

"That depends. May I ask, what is your race?"

"White."

"Caucasian," the social worker writes down. "We have many more black babies than white ones for adoption, and many more white parents seeking to adopt, so the wait is much longer for a white infant. We place babies only with adoptive parents of the same race."

"Could you put our names on the waiting list before the interviews begin?" Bonnie asks.

"No, I'm sorry, we have to assess your eligibility before we can put you on the list," Ms. Winston replies. "Would you like to set up the initial appointment?"

"Yes, I guess so. Are you open on Saturdays?"

"Weekdays only, nine to five," the social worker answers crisply.

"I'm sorry, then, I'll have to call you back," Bonnie says. "My husband and I both have to arrange for time off from work."

"The woman at the adoption agency wasn't very nice," Bonnie says to Larry that evening. "And she's a social worker. I thought social workers were into helping people. This woman sounded like a clerk at the Department of Motor Vehicles."

"Never mind how she sounded. What did she say?" Larry asks.

"She said we have to come down in person for an interview. That's only the beginning. The home study process takes months, she said."

"We've waited this long. What's a few more months?"

"They're only open on weekdays, nine to five. Can you arrange to get off work?"

"Sure. When's the best time for you?"

"As soon as possible is the best time for me," Bonnie answers. They check their calendars, and Bonnie sets up an appointment with the adoption agency for the following week.

In the meantime, the agency mails them a form letter describing the assessment procedures in more detail. The home study process, it says, consists of joint and individual interviews of the applicants and all members of their household. They must provide employment and personal references, and the agency will carry out background checks of state and federal criminal records. When the assessment is completed, the agency then decides whether to approve or reject the couple's application.[4]

Bonnie and Larry arrive at the agency for their appointment with Ms. Winston. The social worker begins by asking for details about their finances, including their income, savings, the mortgage payments on their home, the payments on their auto loan, other installment plans, other indebtedness, and their health and life insurance.

"I see you both work. What are your plans for after you bring the baby home?"

"My wife plans to stay home and care for it," Larry says.

Ms. Winston looks at Bonnie. "Is that correct, Mrs. Roberts?"

"Yes, it is," Bonnie replies, fidgeting.

"Your joint take-home pay is only a little more than you need to cover your monthly expenses. With the added expense of the baby, how do you plan to afford living on only one income?"

"We'll work it out," Larry says. "We've never had any money problems," he adds confidently.

"That may be, but it's our responsibility to make sure every child we place is properly provided for," Ms. Winston says, making notes on the intake form. "We can't leave things to chance, you know," she smiles primly.

The social worker asks about their family background and current family relationships. She informs Larry and Bonnie that before making a home visit, she'll have to meet with each of them separately. She asks them to have their physicians forward copies of their medical records, and requests copies of their employment records for the years since they graduated from college. Consecutive appointments are made for the separate interviews before the couple leaves the agency.

"Whew!" Larry exclaims on the way to the car. "I wonder if that woman was trained by the FBI."

"I don't think she liked all our answers. I'm especially worried about the financial stuff. She made it sound like if I quit my job we can't afford to adopt a baby."

"It's a catch-22," Larry adds. "If you'd said you plan to keep working, then she'd probably have asked how we could afford child care. Or maybe the agency thinks child care isn't good for kids. Who knows? Are there any right answers?"

"I don't know. Let's just be honest with her and hope for the best. Maybe everything will work out."

❁

At their individual interviews, Bonnie and Larry are both surprised by the nature of the questions the social worker asks. Ms. Winston inquires into their philosophy of child rearing and discipline. In her responses,

Bonnie is unsure whether to err on the side of being too permissive or too strict. Larry recalls how his older brother and his wife discipline their children and patterns his answers after their behavior. When the sessions are finished, they compare notes.

"She really gave me the third degree," Larry says.

"Did she question you about corporal punishment?" Bonnie asks.

"Yeah, and a lot more. She asked what I'd do if I caught my child stealing. And using drugs. I think she sneaked some trick questions in there."

"I don't think our answers are any different from most people's. You don't have to be a child psychologist to be able to adopt a baby," Bonnie says hopefully.

"We'll see," Larry replies.

In two weeks Larry gets a call at work from Ms. Winston. "Mr. Roberts, I'd like to arrange a re-interview with you if you don't mind."

"Sure, what's up?"

"The agency has received your medical and employment records, and I have a few additional questions."

Larry is a bit apprehensive when he greets the social worker again. She has some papers spread on the desk in front of her.

"Mr. Roberts, I see here that ten years ago you worked for Ace and Company Products. You worked there for three years, is that correct?"

"That's about right."

"During that time, these records show that you took a three months' leave of absence. Is that correct?"

"Yes."

"Could you please tell me the reason for the leave of absence?"

"It was nothing, really." Larry begins to perspire.

"A note here says 'medical treatment.' There are no further details. What were you treated for, Mr. Roberts?"

"I really don't think that's important now. It was eight years ago."

"It's important to us, Mr. Roberts. Our records have to be complete. I don't see any mention of this treatment in the medical records you sent to us."

"Uh, it was a different doctor."

"I'm sorry, Mr. Roberts, we asked you to send us *all* medical records. Unless our files are complete, we can't process your application."

"Well, I forgot. Can't remember everything, you know. We had to pull a lot of stuff together for this agency. I just didn't remember every little detail from years ago."

"Do you remember the reason for your leave of absence? What kind of medical treatment you had?"

Larry is silent.

"Mr. Roberts, I'm afraid we can't take this any further until you supply all the information we ask for."

"I had a brief episode of posttraumatic stress syndrome. I was referred to a psychiatrist, and he treated me successfully. It never came back." Larry is now perspiring heavily.

"I'll have to ask for that medical record, too. If you could contact the psychiatrist yourself and have him send a copy of your record for that treatment, I will continue with the home study process."

"Okay, I'll do that," Larry says.

Larry and Bonnie hear nothing from the agency for three months. Then one day a letter signed by the associate director informs them that their application for adoption has been rejected on the basis of a finding of "questionable fitness for parenting." No further explanation is provided. Larry is angry and resentful, and Bonnie is despondent. He worries that she will blame him now for their rejection by the agency. She is more desperate than ever, and because of Larry's reaction to the failed attempt at adoption she feels lonelier than before.

One Saturday soon after receiving the disappointing news, Bonnie goes shopping with her sister-in-law. They are riding the escalator to home furnishings when they pass the toddlers' department. Bonnie starts to weep.

"What's wrong?" her sister-in-law asks, fishing a tissue out of her purse.

"Oh Frannie, I can't help it," Bonnie sobs. "Babies and children—it's all I can think about. Larry says I'm obsessing, but I feel so empty inside. I can't stand it!"

"Poor thing. I can sympathize with you. My marriage was so short, we never got around to having kids. But here I am, thirty-three years old, and everyone my age is having babies. It's much worse for you and Larry, though. You're married and really want kids."

"After we were rejected by the adoption agency, Larry and I stopped talking about the problem. Now I'm afraid it's hurting our marriage. Larry always used to be supportive, but now he's so distant."

"Didn't you go to an infertility doctor before you tried adopting?"

"No. Larry didn't want to. We argued about it, and he wouldn't do it."

"Would you like me to talk to him? He usually listens to me. He's had a lot of respect for my ideas since we were teenagers. He told everyone his sister was the only one who understood him."

"Fine with me. I don't know if it will do much good, but it's worth a try."

Frannie talks to Larry, and the conversation has the desired effect. Larry tells Bonnie he's changed his mind, and they make an appointment with their regular doctor, an internist. They feel more comfortable seeing him first and plan to ask for a referral to an infertility specialist.

"I know some very capable people in the field," their doctor says. "I recommend the group practice in the Fecundity Center, located near the medical school. They have at least two board-certified reproductive endocrinologists there."

"Is that what this medical specialty is called?" Bonnie asks.

"Yes, the physicians who go into it are usually 'ob-gyns,' specialists in obstetrics and gynecology. Reproductive endocrinology is a subspecialty that deals with infertility. But before a woman goes for an infertility workup, her husband is usually checked out first. I can refer you to an excellent urologist," the doctor looks at Larry.

"Bonnie can go first. Aren't you willing to do that, Bon?"

"It's not a matter of who's willing," the doctor says. "It's much easier to detect the cause of infertility in the male, and then if a problem is discovered, there's no need for the woman to undergo the more complicated procedures. I can do the basic physical exam on both of you, and if nothing obvious turns up, I'll refer Larry to a urologist for a semen analysis."

"I'm sure there's nothing wrong with me," Larry says.

"You may be right, but we don't know that yet," the doctor replies.

"There's nothing wrong with my sexual performance," Larry insists stridently.

"Larry, it's not about performance," Bonnie says gently.

"Right, it may be physiological. It's not a question of your sexuality," the doctor says.

"It is a question of my manhood, though," Larry replies.

"That's not a good way to think about this," the doctor says. "There may be a minor anatomic anomaly, which can usually be picked up in a physical exam. But the most common cause of male infertility lies in the semen. Basic sperm counts have been performed for many years as a way of evaluating male fertility. Today, there are quite a few new tests, including examination of the volume, pH, and viscosity of seminal fluid, as well as the quantity, motility, and other characteristics of sperm."[5]

Larry is frowning and shakes his head. "I don't know. I never thought of myself as having bad sperm."

"You'll be doing your wife a favor if you go first," the doctor says, switching tactics. "When a woman has a fertility workup, both husband and wife are asked to visit the specialist within a few hours after having intercourse. A sample of your wife's cervical mucus will be taken to determine how sperm interact with the vaginal and cervical environment. After that's done, a more complicated set of tests will have to be performed—"

"All right, all right," Larry agrees impatiently. "I'll go. But what can we do if they find some problem with me?"

"If it's the husband's sperm count that's causing the problem, the standard remedy is to inseminate the wife with sperm from an anonymous donor. You don't have to worry about infectious diseases or known genetic abnormalities," the doctor adds. "These days, a thorough medical history is taken from donors at reputable sperm banks. Sperm are tested for a number of diseases, including the AIDS virus."

"We haven't discussed the possibility of artificial insemination," Bonnie says, looking hesitantly at Larry.

"We'll cross that bridge if and when we come to it," Larry says.

The doctor writes down the name and telephone number of the urologist and hands the paper to Larry. "When you call, just mention that I referred you."

❧

Larry visits the urologist and undergoes the standard infertility workup for men. No abnormalities are found, and Larry is much relieved. He feels that his virility has been proved. The burden of infertility is now placed on Bonnie, who feels that her femininity is challenged. Before she makes an appointment at the Fecundity Center, they visit their internist once again. He explains that infertility workups are often inconclusive, and then goes on to list the array of tests that are done to determine the cause of infertility in women.

"Before I get started with all these tests, we'd like to know what our options would be," Bonnie says.

"That depends on what they find out," the doctor replies.

"I know, but can't you give us a rough idea?" Bonnie asks apprehensively.

"Of course, but remember, this is only a general picture. None of it may apply to you."

Bonnie and Larry nod.

"One of the most common causes of infertility in women is blocked fallopian tubes. If that turns out to be the problem, you could try in vitro fertilization, using your sperm," the doctor looks at Larry and turns back to Bonnie, "and your eggs. Sometimes, though, a woman is unable to produce eggs. In that case, you might choose to use a donor egg, an option similar to donor sperm when there's a problem with the husband's sperm. It's more difficult with a woman, however. You'd have to take hormones. One or more eggs will be extracted from a woman who agrees to be a donor, and then fertilized with your husband's sperm in vitro—you know, in a glass dish. The embryo that results from this process is then implanted in your womb, and if everything is successful, you become pregnant. The Fecundity Center has just started an egg donation program. The program is new, but the physicians are very knowledgeable and skilled in the procedures."

"Sounds like *1984* all over again," Larry says, "and it's already 1994."

"You're thinking of *Brave New World*, dear," Bonnie corrects her husband. She turns to the doctor. "This gives us a lot to think about. Thank you for explaining."

"I haven't explained everything," the doctor cautions. The infertility workup might reveal other possibilities."

"Such as?" Bonnie asks.

"I'll just mention one more, at this point. Your fallopian tubes might be normal, and you might be capable of producing eggs, but sometimes a woman is unable to carry a pregnancy. If there is an uncorrectable abnormality in the uterus, proper implantation can't take place."

"What's the treatment for that?" Bonnie asks.

"When I said 'uncorrectable,' I was referring to a situation for which there's no available treatment." The doctor hesitates. "The only option in that case is to hire a surrogate to carry the baby. I'm not recommending this, you understand, just informing you. I think the Fecundity Center has a surrogacy matching service, but I'm not sure about that. I only know for sure that its medical services are of high quality and reliable."

Bonnie and Larry sit in silence, a bit stunned by this array of possibilities.

"We need some time to think about all this," Bonnie says. "But could you give me a referral to the Fecundity Center for the infertility workup?"

"Certainly," the doctor replies, and writes down the name and telephone number of a reproductive endocrinologist at the clinic.

Bonnie makes an appointment. Her physician is Dr. Furillo, a reproductive endocrinologist specially trained in carrying out diagnostic techniques to identify the cause of infertility in women, extracting eggs from fertile women, and performing in vitro fertilization (IVF) and embryo implantation.

Bonnie's infertility workup is lengthy and costly, but definitive. She has normal ovarian function, but abnormalities in the intrauterine lining make it impossible for an embryo to become implanted, so pregnancy cannot occur. Dr. Furillo offers encouragement to Bonnie, saying that it's better to find a known cause of infertility than to be left in the dark. Furthermore, there is a remedy, although it is not, strictly speaking, a treatment. Elaborating on what the internist has already told the couple, the specialist explains that they can avail themselves of surrogate embryo transfer if they are willing to use a surrogate mother. The Fecundity Center's surrogacy matching service can find a suitable surrogate, properly screened; then, after the couple and the surrogate meet one another, the clinic can draw up a contract. The surrogate would carry the pregnancy, but the baby would be genetically related to Bonnie and Larry, since her egg and his sperm would be used for the fertilization.

"Larry, I'm so confused about all this," Bonnie says when they finally sit down for a long, serious talk. "The doctors explain the medical risks and benefits of the procedures they do, but they don't tell us if these procedures are all right—I mean moral."

"They know about the right and wrong of this stuff. They wouldn't advise us to do something they thought was unethical."

"But these specialists have something to gain. They do in vitro fertilization and get paid for it. And since the Fecundity Center also makes all the arrangements for a surrogate, they get paid for that too. So they're not about to raise ethical questions about artificial reproduction or surrogacy, are they?"

"Not exactly. You're saying they might be unethical? Who can we ask about this stuff?"

"I'm not sure. I know of a pastoral counselor—I'm not sure he does this kind of counseling, but I could ask. He's a minister with a master's degree in counseling psychology."

"How do you know about him?"

"Remember when Charlie and Mary were on the verge of getting divorced? They went to him, and he really helped them a lot."

Bonnie looks in the phone book and finds Rev. Karl Schmidt, M.A., in the yellow pages, under Counseling Services. She makes an appointment for the early evening several days later.

Karl Schmidt is accustomed to counseling couples who are having marital difficulties, but he has never been asked to discuss assisted reproduction with a couple whose problem is infertility.

"I'm not an expert in medicine or biology," the minister begins, "but I do know that these methods are artificial, unnatural."

"Does that make them morally wrong?" Bonnie asks.

"That depends on your religion," Mr. Schmidt answers. "As you know, I'm not a Catholic priest, but I'm certain the Roman Catholic religion disapproves of any artificial means of reproduction. Orthodox Jews are strictly opposed to artificial insemination by an anonymous donor; I'm certain of that, too. Of course, I don't speak officially for my own Protestant denomination, but I think artificial means of reproduction are morally unacceptable because they violate the Natural Law, which is God's law."

"Is that what all Protestants believe?" Larry asks.

"No, it's not. Why, I recently read about a female Episcopal priest who wanted to have a baby but didn't want a husband. I think that's a sin, in and of itself. Anyway, she invited three friends over—please forgive me for what I'm about to tell you, but this lady priest asked these three men (two of them priests, mind you) to masturbate for her so that she could impregnate herself with their sperm."[6]

"Excuse me, Reverend Schmidt, I feel embarrassed talking about this," Bonnie says. "But why did she need three men to give her their sperm?"

"She explained, on national television, in fact, that she wanted several sperm sources so she wouldn't know who the father was and could 'make sure that the child would have an intimate bond to no one but herself.'[7] I find the whole thing abhorrent."

"Tell us more about your own objections, would you, Reverend?" Larry inquires.

"As I said, it's not natural. In vitro fertilization is making life by manufacturing, is it not? Test-tube babies are manufactured. 'Procreation, parenthood, is certainly one of those "courses of action" natural to man, which cannot without violation be disassembled and put together again.'"[8]

"But is everything artificial necessarily bad?" Bonnie asks.

"Why, no," the minister replies. "Artificial means of prolonging life, such as respirators or feeding tubes, are moral goods."

"How can you judge one artificial process to be good and another to be bad, then?" Larry inquires.

" 'The proper objective of medicine is to serve and care for man as a natural object, to help in all our natural "courses of action," to tend the garden of our creation.'[9] Doctors have tried from the earliest times to heal human diseases and to prolong life in accordance with God's wishes. Artificial means of prolonging life are merely an extension of natural means. Take foods and fluids, for one example. Some people argue that artificial nutrition and hydration are medical treatments, and so a patient may refuse them or doctors may withhold them from patients. But the fact that food and fluids are delivered through tubes doesn't make them any the less food and fluids that are basic to life. Regardless of the way they come into the human body, food and fluids are sustenance, part of nature. It is a sin to deny any living person basic nurturance.

"On the other hand," the minister continues, "to create life in a test tube, to take an embryo from a dish and surgically implant it in the uterus of a woman, that's something neither God nor nature ever intended. We are part of an environment that works 'according to its lineaments, according to the functions we discover to be the case in the whole assemblage of natural objects.' "[10]

"Is the fact that it's artificial the only reason you think these means of reproduction are wrong? Are there any other ethical reasons?" Bonnie asks, a touch of skepticism in her voice.

"There is more. 'At stake is the *idea* of the *humanness* of our human life and the meaning of our embodiment, our sexual being, and our relation to ancestors and descendants.'[11] We owe respect to humanity simply because it is humanity, a unique creation of God. But it is not only as God's creatures that we owe respect to humanity. There are also '*the bonds of lineage, kinship, and descent.* To be human means not only to have human form and powers; it means also to have a human context and to be humanly connected.' "[12]

"But Reverend Schmidt, that's just the point. We want children; we want to be humanly connected. Our longing for a baby is part of our human feelings, isn't it?" Bonnie asks with determination.

"Certainly, of course. I understand your desire for children, and I sympathize with your problem of infertility. But all children are God's creatures. Isn't adoption the proper solution to your problem?"

"Unfortunately not," Larry says. "We tried, but we were rejected."

The minister looks a bit suspicious. "A nice young couple like you? May I ask the reason for the rejection? I'm a trained counselor in addition to being a minister, you know. Maybe I can help."

Larry doesn't feel comfortable. "They just rejected us, that's all. I really don't want to talk about it. We came to you to ask about the ethics of assisted reproduction because we're confused. With all due respect, Reverend, we're not looking for counseling for anything else."

"As you wish," the minister replies. "What else can I tell you, then?"

"I think I understand your position about artificial reproduction," Bonnie says. "I guess there isn't anything else."

"I can't think of anything else either," Larry says.

Mr. Schmidt rises. "Well, then, let me add to what I've already said, and tell you that I think these developments mark 'the return of eugenics,' involving 'the manufacture of synthetic children, the fabrication of families, [and] artificial sex.'[13] From the standpoint of ethics, which for me is inseparable from religion, these developments represent one of the moral evils of our time."

❀

"Whew, heavy duty!" Larry exclaims as he starts the car. "That guy sounds pretty dogmatic to me."

"He's religious."

"I don't care how religious he is. I still don't get his point about which artificial things are immoral. Did you understand his answer to my question?"

"Which one?"

"You know, after you asked if everything that's artificial is necessarily wrong."

"Not really," Bonnie replies. "Some of his points were obscure."

"Isn't that what I said?"

"No, you called him dogmatic."

"Well, he was that too. Obscure and dogmatic. What should we do now?"

"I think we should get another opinion. When you go to a surgeon who recommends surgery, you have a right to a second opinion. We can do the same thing in our situation."

"Not a bad idea," Larry says. "But where will we get the opinion? From another minister?"

"I had someone else in mind. A bioethicist."

"A what?"

"A bioethicist. The other afternoon I was listening to a talk show on the radio. The guest was an ethicist in residence at the medical school. I liked what she had to say."

"Was she talking about artificial reproduction?"

"No, the program was on the ethics of withholding artificial food and fluids from dying patients."

"At least it was about artificial something."

"Larry, that's not why I'm suggesting we talk to the ethicist, because she's an expert on artificial everything. What she said made good common sense. And she was clear, not like this minister we just talked to."

"Okay, so give her a call. It shouldn't be too hard to track her down."

❧

Bonnie learns that the ethicist, Teddi Chernacoff, is in the Department of Medical Humanities at the medical school. Professor Chernacoff agrees to meet the couple in her office at 6:00 P.M. later that week. When Bonnie and Larry arrive, she ushers them into a small academic office. The walls are lined with bookshelves, a computer stands on one side of the desk, and the desktop is cluttered with papers.

"Thanks very much for agreeing to see us," Bonnie says. "I know you must be very busy."

"Never too busy for important ethical concerns," the bioethicist replies. "You said on the phone you had some questions about the ethics of assisted reproduction."

"We were hoping you could counsel us about that," Larry says.

"I have to tell you, to start with, that I'm not a counselor. I'm not a psychologist, a social worker, or a specialist in infertility."

"I know, you're an ethicist. I heard you on the radio." Bonnie smiles. "My husband and I thought you could give us some ethical advice."

"I'm reluctant to call it advice," Chernacoff says. "Ethicists don't normally tell people what to do. That's the job of *moralists*. What I can do for you is clarify the issues, explain the ethical problems some people have found with assisted reproduction, and sort out arguments for and against IVF, egg donation, surrogacy, and other methods. But the decision about whether to use any of these methods is entirely up to you."

"Could you clear up a question about whether artificial methods are ethically wrong?"

"I could begin with that point, if you like. This objection to reproductive technologies is sometimes made by religious ethicists. They try to make a moral distinction between what is 'natural' and what is 'artificial.' But I think it's impossible to defend that distinction for the purpose of drawing ethical conclusions. Just think of the numerous advances science and technology have contributed to so many spheres of human life. That leads to a puzzle about why reproductive techniques should be condemned as unethical simply on the ground that they are artificial.

"I find it curious, for example, that opponents of artificial methods of reproduction are among the most enthusiastic supporters of technological means of sustaining and prolonging life. These people endorse the use of respirators (artificial breathing machines), dialysis machines (artificial kidneys), and other life supports. In fact, many of these same people are opposed to withholding or withdrawing artificial food and fluids, even from patients who are near death."

"We spoke with someone who took that position," Bonnie says. "He's a minister."

"Is he a Catholic?" Chernacoff asks.

"No, Protestant," Larry answers.

"I didn't mean to single out the Roman Catholic religion," Chernacoff quickly adds. "I make the same point about any religion. Even if the teachings of a particular religion bind its adherents, those who are devout believers in its teachings, nothing follows concerning the morality of the practice for nonbelievers. A religion may impose duties and prohibitions on its believers that are morally neutral to others. Even if a particular religion condemns a societal practice or personal behavior, that doesn't make it morally wrong or even ethically controversial."

"The minister we spoke to said that ethics and religion are inseparable."

"That's one viewpoint. Understandably, it's the viewpoint of theologians and the clergy. But in addition to religious ethics, secular ethics is a legitimate field. Secular ethics is guided by a number of fundamental principles, and many highly moral people don't take their ethics from a religious system."

"It's a relief to hear that," Larry says.

"Well, just to finish the point we were discussing," Chernacoff resumes, "the distinction between what is natural and what is artificial is hard to draw conceptually, and even more problematic when we're trying to determine what is ethical and what is unethical. To base the ethical rightness or wrongness of the new reproductive technologies on their artificiality is to make an arbitrary judgment, which can't stand up to ethical scrutiny."

"Are you saying there aren't any ethical problems at all with artificial reproduction?" Bonnie asks.

"No, I haven't said that. At least not yet," Chernacoff smiles. "But I suggest we don't use the term 'artificial,' so we can avoid the kinds of objections we've been talking about. We can call it 'assisted reproduction' or 'third-party collaboration,' if you like. I prefer the term 'new reproductive practices,' myself. It doesn't beg any ethical questions, and it's probably more accurate in describing the range of activities we have in mind. Anyway, to get back to the ethical issues.

"Some people raise objections similar to those typically made against abortion. I think it's very important to resist such comparisons, but certain groups have made the analogy, as follows. Human life begins at conception. That's when personhood begins. Now IVF typically involves fertilizing more eggs than doctors intend to implant. If a fertilized ovum has moral standing from the very moment of fertilization, then whether an embryo is destroyed in the process of abortion or as a spare embryo, there's no ethical difference. The objection is the same in both cases. It's taking an innocent life."

"Do you believe that?" Bonnie asks.

"My personal beliefs aren't important here; it's what you believe that counts," Chernacoff answers. "But if you want to know what I believe, I favor a woman's right to have an abortion. I would argue that embryos do not have moral standing, and the same factors that make it ethically permissible to terminate a pregnancy make it ethically permissible to destroy unimplanted embryos, if that turns out to be necessary."

"We believe in abortion rights, too." Larry says. "So I guess we have to accept your argument."

"You don't have to," Chernacoff responds. "But it would be ethically consistent. There are other questions pertaining to embryos, especially since they can now be frozen, but at this early stage of your thinking I don't think those questions are relevant."

"Could you tell us what they are, though? We'd like to have everything spelled out, so we can think about it," Bonnie says.

"Okay, briefly then, here are the questions. Once embryos are frozen, to whom do they belong? The couple whose biological product they are? The clinic that does the IVF? What if the couple disagrees about whether the embryos should be destroyed? What if they get divorced, and their frozen embryos are still in storage? If a couple plans no future pregnancies and the clinic wishes to offer them to other infertile couples, should the original couple lose the right to decide about the fate of the embryos?"

"Jeez!" Larry exclaims. "I had no idea we'd have to deal with all these things. It's mind-boggling!"

"Could you say something about the ethics of surrogacy before we're through?" Bonnie asks tentatively, as she notices Chernacoff taking a peek at her watch.

"Sure. In the first place, surrogacy is often classified under the heading of new reproductive technologies. But only a small minority of surrogacy arrangements involve the truly novel techniques of egg retrieval, IVF, and implantation; most employ the long-established technique of artificial insemination, which isn't really new. The first pregnancy reported from artificial insemination goes back to 1799, and artificial insemination by donor started in the 1890s.[14] In fact, even the idea that it involves technology may be suspect. It's often referred to as 'turkey-baster technology.'

"The temporary use of the womb of a woman who will carry the pregnancy but isn't intended to raise the child, however, *is* a new reproductive arrangement. For a number of reasons, it deserves ethical scrutiny. Some people argue that surrogacy is a form of exploitation of women. Additional questions have been raised about the commercial aspects. Other concerns relate to the children who are born of surrogacy arrangements: can it be harmful to them in any way? And still other ethical and legal worries focus on surrogacy contracts and possible disputes between the contracting parties. I'm afraid I don't have more time now to go into these issues with you, but I do have a suggestion. We have a Task Force on Reproduction, appointed by the state legislature, which meets once a month, and the meetings are open to the public. Why don't you consider attending one or more of the meetings? I sit on the task force, along with some other members of this community. We meet in the state capital, but that's only a forty-five-minute drive from here. I think you'd learn a lot, and there's much food for thought."

"Would we understand what goes on?"

"Absolutely. The usual format is to have short presentations by members of the task force, followed by discussion and often heated debates. Sometimes we have a guest speaker on a special topic. The presentations are all designed to educate, since everyone's a layperson in everyone else's field."

"Thank you for telling us," Bonnie says.

"Yes, thanks a lot," Larry chimes in. "Now—uh—how much do we owe you, Professor Chernacoff?"

"Oh, you don't owe me anything!" she says. "I consider this part of my work as an educator in the field of bioethics."

"Don't ethicists usually charge for consultations?" Larry asks. "After all, we paid the reverend we went to see."

"He's a counselor, Larry. Professor Chernacoff is a bioethicist."

"Some ethicists do charge for their consultations," Chernacoff says. "I might, in other circumstances. For example, if I'm asked by a city or state government for an ethics consultation, I receive a fee for preparing a document, such as an ethical analysis of a case. But this was just an informal meeting to answer some of your questions and clarify some ethical issues. I think it would be unethical for me to get paid for that.

"Now there's one last thing. For more information about all this, you might call the local chapter of Resolve—that's a nationwide support group for infertile people."

❀

"She didn't really give us much advice," Larry says after their meeting with Teddi Chernacoff.

"She said she wasn't going to give advice, didn't she?" Bonnie says defensively.

"I guess so. But I agree with what you said; she states things clearly. The stuff about what's artificial and what's natural was really good. We can lay that problem to rest."

"What about the embryos, though?" Bonnie asks. "She gave us her views on that, but said we have to decide what we believe about destroying embryos. I'm still not too sure."

"Didn't she say if we're in favor of abortion there's no reason to be concerned about destroying embryos?"

"She said something like that. But she insisted that it's our beliefs, not hers, that matter."

"What do you suggest?"

"Maybe we should look for another consultation. Someone who can tell us more about embryos."

"Do you have anyone in mind?"

"Not really. Maybe another religious counselor, from a different religion."

"No!" Larry insists. "I see no point at all in that."

"Then I'm going to call that Resolve organization she mentioned. The more we can find out, the better we'll be able to come to the right decision."

"The way I see it, the more we find out, the more complicated it gets," Larry says.

❖

Bonnie telephones the Resolve office the next morning. An earnest woman with a pleasant voice tells her that the mission of the organization is to supply information about infertility, make referrals to physicians and clinics that provide services, and sponsor support groups for infertile couples. The organization encourages couples to look at all available options before choosing surrogacy but considers surrogacy an appropriate option. Resolve takes the position that freedom of choice is a value that requires continued legality of surrogacy arrangements. The woman says she will send Bonnie some literature.

Bonnie and Larry learn from the material they receive in the mail that Resolve, Inc., is a nonprofit organization founded in Boston in 1973. The founder, Barbara Menning, was a woman diagnosed as infertile who found herself in need of emotional support and quality medical care. Ms. Menning met with friends and acquaintances who shared a similar plight, and in 1978 she was successful in obtaining a small family-planning grant that enabled her to set up a small office and train family planning staff. By 1981 the organization had grown to thirty-five Resolve chapters across the United States, run by volunteers, and by 1988 forty-seven affiliated chapters were offering monthly programs, formal support groups, counseling, and medical information. The national office maintains a list of specialists throughout the country, to which members are referred, and distributes literature to local chapters and members.[15]

The information packet includes a personal account written by a woman who had suffered the consequences of infertility for years. Her story describes infertility as a "silent and devastating" condition, something "you wish you could die from." She had undergone many surgical procedures and spent two years in an IVF program; twelve embryos were implanted, but all attempts failed. The woman and her husband were not candidates for adoption. Her tale tells of suffering through family births and those of friends. Infertility consumed her days and nights. Her feelings ranged from anger to grief to self-pity, then more anger.[16] Bonnie empathizes with the woman and reads on.

Six years earlier the infertile woman had contracted with a surrogate to produce a child. The woman chosen—who was not "shanghaied off the street," the narrator wrote—was inseminated with the sperm of the infertile woman's husband. Her medical bills were covered, and she was paid for her time and effort and for the risks of the pregnancy and childbirth. This was the last hope for the infertile couple to have a child of their own, and it worked. In fact, the experience of everyone involved was so positive that the surrogate volunteered to serve again in that capacity for the same couple.[17]

❀

"This literature convinces me that surrogate motherhood is a good thing," Bonnie says. "Resolve sounds like a respectable organization."

"That may be, but they only present one side of the picture," Larry replies. "There must be another side, or else there wouldn't be so much controversy over this surrogacy business. Let's not get sucked in too quickly."

"Don't you think we should go to one of the Resolve support group meetings?"

"I think we should take the professor's suggestion and go to the government committee meeting. What did she call it, the Task Force on Procreation?"

"Reproduction."

"Yeah, that's it. Let's go to the next meeting and see what we can learn."

"I'm ready."

Debating Assisted Reproduction

Bonnie and Larry slide into seats at the rear of the conference room just as Maura O'Brien, chair of the Task Force on Reproduction, is calling the meeting to order. Ms. O'Brien, an attorney, asks for approval of the minutes of the last meeting. She then announces that the newly appointed chair of a similar task force in a neighboring state is present and suggests that the task force members introduce themselves briefly to the visitor.

"I'm Father Timothy Reardon, professor of theology at St. Matthews College."

"I'm LeRoy Johnson, state assemblyman."

"My name is Andrea Goldwoman, and I represent WARO, Women against Reproductive Oppression."

"Good evening. John Ward. I'm pastor of the First Methodist Church."

"Dr. Roberta Bernstein, psychologist."

"I'm Vera Rodriguez, a nurse at Mercy Hospital."

"Dr. Anthony Romano. I'm on the faculty at the College of Medicine in the Department of Obstetrics and Gynecology. My specialty is reproductive endocrinology."

"My name is Jeanne Lodge. I'm a community representative on the task force."

"And I'm Teddi Chernacoff, bioethicist at the College of Medicine."

"Bill Ackerman, lawyer working with the task force."

"Tod Nielsen, practicing attorney."

"Thanks, everyone. The topic for tonight's meeting is the status of the embryo as it relates to new reproductive technologies. We've asked several task force members to prepare brief presentations to get the discussion started. Let's begin with Dr. Romano."

"Okay. Maura asked me to say a few things about some of the biological and technical issues, so we have a common background for our discussion. I'm sure you all learned about fertilization and early development of the embryo in your basic biology course, but let me review briefly.

"In the natural setting, fertilization of the female egg by the male sperm normally takes place in the oviduct. The wall of the egg is penetrated by the sperm, and genetic material from sperm and egg unite to form a new cell, termed a 'zygote.' The process of cell division then begins, and in the earliest stages the group of cells is called a 'conceptus.' The timing of these developing stages isn't known with precision, but as cell division continues over the next three or four days the conceptus becomes a 'blastocyst.' Then comes the process of implantation as the blastocyst attaches to the lining of the uterus. This occurs about six or seven days after the woman's ovulation.

"Now we come to an important point that may appear to be mere semantics but is critical for determining the status of the embryo. The preferred term for the mass of dividing cells, including the blastocyst up to fourteen days after fertilization, is 'preembryo.' Some people continue to speak loosely of the entity at this stage as an 'embryo,' but biologically, that's inaccurate. This is because it's impossible at this stage to distinguish between the cells in the outer wall that eventually become the placenta and the internal cells that become the fetus. So we use the term 'preembryo' for this early stage when all the cells are more or less equivalent. The next critical development occurs at about fourteen days after fertilization, when the 'primitive streak' appears. This is the group of cells that indicates the beginning of the nervous system. Then, between the end of the second week and the eighth or ninth week, we have the embryonic period, a significant stage of development. The transition from embryo to fetus occurs at eight to nine weeks after fertilization."[1]

"Dr. Romano, may I ask a question at this point?" Jeanne Lodge inquires tentatively.

"Of course, go right ahead."

"This may sound stupid, but when, exactly, does conception take place?"

"It's not stupid at all, it's a very good question," Dr. Romano replies. "In fact, it's a matter of some controversy. One leading authority has argued that conception 'cannot be thought of as only fertilization. The continuum of the reproductive process includes meiosis before fertilization, implantation (a process taking several days), and several steps necessary for the proper development of the embryo.'[2] Our ability to do in vitro fertilization shows quite clearly where sharp lines can and cannot be drawn. A woman's egg can be fertilized in a dish, but obviously, she is not pregnant until the preembryo becomes attached to her uterus."

"You'll probably be surprised to learn that one court ruled otherwise," Bill Ackerman interjects. "In a 1983 case challenging the Illinois law pertaining to in vitro fertilization, a court accepted the notion that a woman undergoing IVF is pregnant from the moment her egg is fertilized, despite the fact that the fertilization has taken place outside her body."[3]

Andrea Goldwoman nearly jumps out of her chair. "That's ridiculous! Calling a woman pregnant because her fertilized eggs are sitting in a dish! I suppose the fetal police will be after her if she drinks a margarita while the extracorporeal conceptus is alive."

"Don't be so quick to condemn it, Andrea," Bill Ackerman rejoins. "The implication of the court ruling is that any decision about disposal—especially destruction—may not be made without the woman's consent."[4]

"It still seems ridiculous."

Anthony Romano questions: "How can a judge make a ruling on a purely medical matter? 'According to its medical definition, pregnancy begins at the completion of implantation of the embryo in the woman's womb. This definition has been adopted by the American College of Obstetricians and Gynecologists. The Committee on Medical Aspects of Human Reproduction of the International Federation of Gynecology and Obstetrics unanimously agreed that "pregnancy is only established with the implantation of the fertilized ovum."' "[5]

"Tony, there's room for dispute over whether definitions *are* a purely medical matter," Teddi Chernacoff intervenes. "A definition must be consistent with scientific facts, but as knowledge is expanded, definitions can be refined and even altered. Before current knowledge of the reproductive process was available, the terms 'conception' and 'fertilization' could have been used interchangeably. Whether to expand or change a definition in light of new knowledge requires a decision; it isn't purely a matter of scientific discovery."

Bill Ackerman adds, "Yes, but in the case I referred to, *Smith v. Hartigan*, the judge didn't base his ruling on new scientific knowledge. That was a political decision, designed to give control over the embryos to the woman whose eggs were fertilized in vitro. So the judge determined that she should be called pregnant."

"That contradicts generally accepted medical practice in IVF programs. In every program I know of, 'pregnancy is considered to begin at the completion of implantation of an egg fertilized outside the womb,'" Anthony Romano asserts.[6]

LeRoy Johnson addresses a question to Dr. Romano. "Then there's no problem with the disposal of embryos—I guess I should say *pre*embryos—that never get implanted? I seem to recall a few years ago an attempt by the United States Congress to declare that human life begins at conception. Wasn't there a proposed constitutional amendment to that effect? And also a bill introduced into Congress? But if you're saying that conception begins at the time of implantation, then there should be no ethical problem about destroying a preembryo or embryo that's not implanted, right?"

"No, that's not quite right," Father Reardon interjects. "Some older language refers to 'the moment of conception,' but the Vatican's 'Instruction on Respect for Human Life' issued in 1987 uses different terminology. It speaks of 'the dignity of newly begotten life.' And even back in 1974, the Vatican declaration on abortion stated, 'Right from fertilization is begun the adventure of a human life.'[7] We can't escape the moral issue by verbal sleight of hand. Reverence for human life—"

The chairperson interrupts: "Father Reardon, you're our next speaker. You'll have plenty of time to state your position fully. I think we should let Dr. Romano finish his presentation before we plunge into debate. Please, let's limit the discussion during the speakers' presentations to factual questions only. Would you resume, please, Dr. Romano?"

"Okay, where was I?"

"Before Ms. Lodge asked her question about when conception takes place, you had just finished describing the transition from embryo to fetus at eight or nine weeks. And then Mr. Johnson asked about destroying unimplanted preembryos."

"Yes. In answer to LeRoy, I can only tell you what has become accepted practice. 'In the United States, the loss of fertilized eggs in in vitro fertilization programs is accepted and is not considered abortion.'[8] I think that's all I need to go into about early development through the embryonic stage. Let me turn next to IVF and cryopreservation, since we'll be discussing ethical issues surrounding freezing, storing, and disposing of unimplanted embryos.

"Remember I said that during the earliest phase of development—up to the point where more than sixteen cells exist—all the cells of the blastocyst are roughly equivalent. Following in vitro fertilization the preembryo is transferred to the uterine cavity. This is done at the two- to sixteen-cell stage. That's also the time at which the preembryo would be frozen. So you see, there's no question of whether or not this is an embryo. These preembryos consist of fewer than sixteen cells, and at the time they are either frozen or extra ones are discarded, they are well under fourteen days old."

Tod Nielsen queries: "Which factor matters here from an ethical point of view—the number of cells or the age of the embryo, or preembryo?"

"I'm a physician; you'll have to ask the ethicist that question. I can say, though, that the two are interrelated. The number of cells marks the stage of development, and development occurs over specific periods of time."

"May I say a word here?" Teddi Chernacoff looks at the task force chairperson.

"No, not yet. Let's let Dr. Romano finish before we get into the moral status of the embryo."

"I'm almost through. We don't need to go into the technical details of oocyte retrieval and IVF now, since we're really interested in the fertilized ovum. Before cryopreservation was perfected, and even today in many IVF centers, the practice has been to attempt fertilization of more eggs than are intended for implantation. This is necessary because not all attempts succeed. We could, of course, choose to fertilize only the exact number of eggs we intend to implant, so the problem of discarding unused preembryos could theoretically be eliminated. But practically speaking, the technique of cryopreservation has enabled us to avoid the problem of discarding unused, unimplanted embryos."

"Dr. Romano," Rev. John Ward asks, "why don't you freeze the woman's eggs? Wouldn't that solve the problem?"

"Right now that's not technically feasible. Although a few births from oocytes that had been frozen have been recorded in Australia and West Germany, the practice of freezing oocytes is very rare. The unfertilized egg is extremely susceptible to damage from the present techniques of cryopreservation."[9]

"Doesn't freezing the embryos only push the problem back for a while?" Tod Nielsen questions. "After all, you have to thaw them sometime. Or can they be frozen indefinitely?"

"First of all, current data show that half of all frozen embryos will not survive thawing even if they're thawed soon after freezing. Second, the process is only a few years old. We don't have enough accumulated data to indicate with any certainty how long preembryos can remain frozen and survive."

"Well, then, you have a problem right there," Vera Rodriguez observes. "Those embryos would presumably survive if they were all implanted instead of being frozen, so freezing them doubles the risk that they'll die."

"I'm sorry, we seem to be getting into substance again," Maura O'Brien rules.

"Okay, but just let me respond to Vera before I turn to my final topic; then I'm through. It's not quite true to say that if all preembryos were implanted they would all survive. Only a fourth to a third of all conceptions in the natural setting—that is, in the woman's body—go on to become live-born infants. The rest are lost at some point between the time of fertilization and the end of pregnancy. Accurate figures are difficult to obtain, because loss of preembryos is especially high soon after fertilization, before it has been determined that a woman is pregnant.[10] So you see, even without artificial means of reproduction, there's a natural loss of the products of conception."

"With all due respect, Dr. Romano, isn't it a bit unseemly to speak of 'products of conception'?" Mr. Ward interjects. "It sounds like you're talking about manufactured objects."

"I'm using the standard terminology in my field. Maybe that language was introduced in order to neutralize the feelings and values associated with performing abortions. It's in that context that we tend to speak of emptying the uterine cavity of the products of conception."

"When you sterilize the language, you harden the heart," Father Reardon intones.

Dr. Romano resumes. "Actually, this brings me to the final point of my presentation. I just want to mention one further consequence of medical advances in treating infertility. When we diagnose the cause of a woman's infertility, it's not always necessary to embark on IVF or one of the other new technologies. Some women respond well to infertility drugs, and this would be the first thing we'd try. But the most commonly prescribed fertility drug, clomiphene citrate, carries a risk of multiple gestation. This is true also of other drugs used to induce ovulation.[11] Once you get more than two or at most three fetuses, there's a risk of premature delivery, low birthweight, and pregnancy complications to the mother as well—gestational diabetes, toxemia, and others.[12] The usual remedy is to recommend a pregnancy reduction."

"A *what*? I thought there was no such thing as being 'a little bit pregnant,'" LeRoy Johnson comments.

"Another term used is 'selective termination' of a certain number of the fetuses," Dr. Romano continues. "It's done only during the first trimester."

"So we are talking about abortion here," Father Reardon asserts.

"Uh oh, this is a hot one," LeRoy Johnson says. "I was hoping we'd be able to talk about new reproductive technologies without getting into abortion. We've spent enough time on that already in the legislature, and I guess we're going to be forced right back into it."

Maura O'Brien intervenes. "I think it's time to turn to Father Reardon's presentation. We'll have plenty of time for discussion after the four formal presentations. Father Reardon."

"I think most of you know what I'm going to say. I'm a Roman Catholic priest and a professor of Catholic theology. I adhere to the Vatican 'Instruction on Procreation,' not simply because I'm a good Catholic but also because I believe it's morally correct. As a fellow priest has observed, 'Reverence for the human person has traditionally been linked to the moment of conception.'[13] The zygote, or the union of two sex cells, is worthy of being considered a 'person.' This traditional Catholic position is supported by modern science, which in this century has been able to verify that the fusion of sperm and egg initiates life and that the union of sperm and egg forms forty-six chromosomes, a unique genetic individual.

"The embryo must be regarded for its own particular worth, identity, and vocation. Even those brought into being 'in vitro' are living gifts of God, possessing dignity and rights. But it is an unquestioned doctrine of the faith that 'the beginning of individual human life must be situated within the conjugal union of husband and wife. . . . The embryo . . . has the *right to be conceived* and *born* in the unique setting of the marital bond where the parents provide for and respect its life from the start.'[14]

"The Vatican 'Instruction on Respect for Human Life in Its Origin and on the Dignity of Procreation' asserts the rights of the preborn: to be conceived, carried in the womb, brought into the world and brought up within marriage. It is contrary to our faith to substitute for or replicate the act of procreation with scientific procedures. Those who suffer from infertility deserve compassion, and we must provide love, support, and pastoral care. The intervention of science, with its artificial means of reproduction, diminishes the dignity of the child to be born. The Instruction reminds us of the true meaning of marriage and procreation. A personalist view of the human body and an affirmation of human dignity at all stages of life are the teachings it emphasizes. These teachings preclude the intervention of science into the procreative process. This is not because life born of human lovemaking is *better* life. Rather, it is marked with 'the ineradicable character of an identity inseparable from the name and the promise of human love.'[15]

"Human procreation is distinctive and sacred because of 'its insistence that new life—a new, individual, human life—is more than the "sum of the procreative partners." The unitive and procreative are inseparably—even if mysteriously—linked in the bond of husband and wife.'[16]

"Thus our official theological teachings prohibit all forms of artificial insemination, in vitro fertilization, and surrogate motherhood. These practices are morally illicit and cannot be justified by the desire to procreate. Roman Catholic theology is not opposed to modern science, however. When science is able to enhance the possibility of procreation through normal conjugal relations, such interventions are morally licit. An example is gamete intrafallopian transfer, or GIFT."[17]

"Could you explain that procedure, Father Reardon?"

"I'd prefer to let Dr. Romano explain it."

Maura O'Brien signals Dr. Romano to go ahead.

"Gamete intrafallopian transfer is a method of treating infertility in which sperm and eggs are directly transferred into the fallopian tubes. Fertilization occurs in the fallopian tubes, just as it does in normal sexual intercourse.[18] Do you want me to say more about this procedure, Ms. O'Brien?"

"No, unless anyone has any questions, I think we should focus on issues relevant to Father Reardon's presentation. Please continue, Father."

"Before concluding, I want to say a bit more about the treatment of embryos. It should be perfectly obvious from everything I've said so far that destruction of embryos is illicit. Even the freezing of embryos is contrary to our teaching. Just as discarding human embryos manifests 'in the extreme the unraveling of conjugal dignity,' so too does freezing them. 'Human persons have the right to be brought into being and sustained by parental rather than technological solicitude. Only the former provides the personal environment where the child is fully vested with human rights and dignity and is protected from being compromised or objectified even by the desire to have a child.' [19] We need always to keep in the forefront of our minds the centrality of human dignity at all stages of life."

"Thank you very much, Father Reardon. I'm sure we all have a better understanding of the position of the Roman Catholic church, especially the theological basis for opposing artificial modes of reproduction. Does anyone have any questions for Father Reardon? Yes, Mr. Johnson."

"You didn't mention it in your presentation, but I seem to recall that when the Vatican issued its 'Instruction on Procreation,' its contents were intended not only for Catholics but as a broad public policy that should apply to everyone. Am I right about that?"

"Yes, that's correct," Father Reardon acknowledges.

"Well, I have a problem with that. In this country, at least, the constitutional separation of church and state doesn't permit the Catholic church or any other religion to dictate a doctrine binding on all citizens."

Father Reardon replies, "The Church does not urge the imposition of the views stated in the Instruction on persons of other faiths *because* they are the views of the Catholic Church. No, it is because they are believed to be morally correct views, prohibiting what is morally illicit for all human persons. The dignity of Protestant and Jewish embryos is at stake here, as well as persons conceived by Catholic parents."

Tod Nielsen whispers to Bill Ackerman. "Is there such a thing as a 'Protestant embryo'?"

Ackerman whispers back: "I don't know about Protestant embryos, but I guess there can be Jewish ones. A child born of a Jewish mother is Jewish."

"Yeah, but we're talking about embryos. They're not born yet. Besides, what if the embryo is implanted in a non-Jewish surrogate mother and the egg came from another woman who is Jewish? Is the embryo Jewish or not?"

The chairperson addresses the whispering attorneys. "Would you like to share your conversation with the rest of us?"

"I'm sorry," Tod replies. "It was a small point of detail."

"All right, Mr. Johnson, do you want to pursue that line of questioning with Father Reardon?"

"No, not at the moment. But I still have some doubts about the issue of religious doctrine and public policy."

"That issue may come up again, so let's table it for the moment. Our next presentation is by Andrea Goldwoman, who'll give us the feminist perspective on some of these issues. But first, let's take a ten-minute break."

❀

When the task force reassembles, Andrea Goldwoman begins. "The world is a political struggle between men and women, with men constantly seeking to dominate women by inventing, developing, and medicalizing ever new approaches to domination. As with any new development, technological or political, we need to ask: Where will all this lead?

" 'In evaluating the new reproductive technologies, a principal concern of feminist ethics is to see how each innovation fits into existing patterns of oppression. Technology is not neutral, so it is important to consider who controls it, who benefits from it, and how each activity is likely to affect women's subordinate status in society.'[20] Some of my feminist sisters argue that new reproductive technologies have been created and are being used by male medical scientists and clinicians for their own personal glory and financial reward. Even those of us who don't go quite that far still believe that a likely result will be a fragmentation of women's functions into egg donor, womb donor, and social mother, threatening to erode the power of motherhood.

"Lest you think my organization is among the extremists of feminist thinking on these matters, I can assure you it's not. An international coalition that goes by the acronym FINRRAGE—Feminist International Network of Resistance to Reproductive and Genetic Engineering—opposes reproductive technology in general and IVF techniques specifically. Members believe that these represent the newest effort by men to control women. They contend that new reproductive technologies are a horrifying extension of patriarchal control over and violence against women."

Tod Nielsen whispers to Bill Ackerman: "She sounds like something straight out of the sixties."

Ackerman replies, "She wasn't so strident until fifteen years ago. That was when she joined up with the radical feminists and changed her name."

Goldwoman ignores the whispering and continues. "Many people— especially bioethicists—claim that the new reproductive technologies don't present any new ethical problems. They are just old ethical problems dressed up in new technological clothing. I disagree. Let me turn briefly to the feminist framework that explains the new and unique problems we feminists see.

"First and foremost, we view reproductive technologies as a product of existing social patterns and values. Since these existing social patterns are patriarchal and oppressive of women, their products and values will also be patriarchal and oppressive of women. A good example is the structure of medical practice and its role in a patriarchal society. 'There is abundant evidence that current medical practice, like its historical predecessors, constitutes a powerful social institution that contributes to the oppression of women.' In particular, 'there is a clear pattern of ever increasing medical control over the various aspects of women's reproductive lives. Menstruation, pregnancy, delivery, lactation, childbearing, abortion, and menopause have already been subjected to medical control.'[21]

"A feminist analysis requires looking at things contextually. Only by understanding the context can we hope to make an appraisal of any new social, scientific, or technological development. This is where a feminist analysis differs from bioethics. Mainstream medical ethics, as done by so-called bioethicists, is an abstract exercise. It fails to attend to the contextual details and is therefore a flawed enterprise. The relevant context here, of course, is the broad political context of reproduction in our society.[22]

"I have two additional subjects to talk about now. The first is a feminist analysis of other medical technologies, those used in prenatal screening; the second is the feminist position on surrogacy. I'll begin with prenatal screening, which includes the possibility of selecting a child's sex. This technique enables people to choose not to have babies with undesired characteristics. Radical feminists who oppose the use of prenatal screening are not out to narrow the choices open to women. Instead, we are concerned about the terrible consequences likely to result. These consequences will be bad not only for women but for disabled persons and, ultimately, society in general.

"Our first assumption is that more women will choose to have boy babies rather than girl babies, or, at least, they would choose to have boys first. The results would then be an imbalance of the male-female ratio, or a preponderance of male firstborn children. Since firstborn children have been found to be more successful or more dominant than subsequently born children, women as a group would suffer from the practice of prenatal sex selection. Our second assumption is that women who decide not to abort a fetus that is shown by prenatal screening to have a mental or physical disability will have greater financial and caretaking burdens.[23] We can predict with some confidence that society will find a way to punish these women for not availing themselves of genetic screening and making what society holds to be the 'right' choice. The negative eugenic possibilities—"

Ms. O'Brien interrupts the presentation at this point.

"Ms. Goldwoman, everything you've said up to now is relevant to the topic of this evening's meeting. But I'm afraid that prenatal diagnosis, sex selection, and negative eugenics are beyond the scope of our discussion here, and even beyond the charge to this task force. I know you have more to say about surrogacy, but that will be the topic of our task force meeting next month. May I ask you please to reserve your comments about surrogacy till then? You'll have enough time on the agenda to present your prepared remarks at that meeting. In order to have time left for general discussion, I'd like to turn now to Mr. Ackerman's presentation on the legal status of the embryo."

Andrea Goldwoman nods her assent. Teddi Chernacoff waves her hand insistently and is recognized by the chair.

"I know we're supposed to hold our substantive comments until after all the formal presentations are finished, but I have an important procedural point to make about Andrea's presentation."

"Go ahead."

"Andrea, I respect your ideological commitment, and I would agree that you've accurately stated the radical feminist viewpoint. But I do think that a balanced presentation to the task force of feminist views should include other positions besides the radical feminist one. It is only fair to point out that there is another group of feminists, the 'liberal feminists.' This group argues that new reproductive technologies such as in vitro fertilization and embryo replacement and transfer will benefit women, since they extend reproductive choices and freedoms.[24] So long as women retain the right *not* to use them, liberal feminists contend that there is nothing wrong with these developments. Feminists don't all speak with one voice when it comes to new reproductive technologies, or even human reproduction more generally."

Noting that the chair does not attempt to halt her comment, Chernacoff continues.

"Two leading ethical perspectives both support the permissibility of using these methods to assist reproduction. The first perspective focuses on the consequences. There is no question about the fact that the use of these technologies enhances the lives and contributes to the happiness of many women. The misery of childlessness and the pain of infertility are relieved by these advances in reproductive endocrinology. So, if we focus on the consequences of using reproductive technologies, it is evident that they produce more happiness than unhappiness.

"As everyone here is aware, this utilitarian argument wouldn't be compelling if anyone's rights were being violated. But nothing Andrea said in support of the radical feminist viewpoint suggested that the rights of women are in jeopardy. To the contrary, I think it can be argued that from the point of view of human rights—an alternative way of looking at ethical issues—women's procreative liberty is enhanced by these developments. Women who choose to avail themselves of these technologies are exercising their autonomy. Their right to reproductive freedom is enlarged by creating opportunities that were unavailable to them before.

"Sometimes the ethical perspective based on the consequences of actions yields a different conclusion from an ethical analysis primarily concerned with the rights of individuals. But since both ethical approaches can be used to justify new reproductive practices, I find it hard to accept the radical feminist critique. This leads me to conclude not only that these reproductive technologies are ethically permissible but that it is ethically desirable to make them available to as many women or couples as may want them. As long as no women are being coerced into using them, and when they give fully informed consent, then no ethical barriers exist."

Andrea Goldwoman's face flushes and her eyes narrow. "You've treated us to the standard liberal account. That's just what's wrong with mainstream bioethics. It's preoccupied with rights and duties, and especially with autonomy. What you call 'women's choices' are simply the products of false consciousness.[25] And informed consent is an illusion, because it rests on an abstract notion of autonomy, divorced from the context of social and political reality."

Jeanne Lodge speaks up. "I think I'm supposed to represent the community here, and I just want to say that the radical feminists Andrea Goldwoman referred to don't speak for all women. Personally, I don't know any women who take that line. I've been to women's support groups; I've attended meetings of the local chapter of NOW; and I have many women friends of different ages. I don't know a single one who talks that way or who thinks that women are being coerced into using these technologies by their husbands, their doctors, or whomever."

"It's the whole society, along with its acceptance of the medical model," Andrea begins again. "Can't you see that these technologies are exploitive? They feed on the idea that infertility and childlessness are abnormalities that make women valueless."

Maura O'Brien is firm. "We really must go on to the next presentation by Bill Ackerman. I think this exchange of views has been useful, and it does underscore Teddi's point that feminists don't all speak with one voice. I'm sure we'll get into this again when we have our discussion of surrogacy. For now, let's turn to Mr. Ackerman's presentation on the legal status of the embryo."

"Thanks, Maura. When I began researching this topic, I came across much more material than I thought I would. Just to give some idea of the scope of concern at the policy level, I learned that between 1979 and 1987 at least eighty-five statements on the new reproductive technologies were prepared by committees representing at least twenty-five countries throughout the world.[26] These committee statements covered everything from in vitro fertilization, surrogate motherhood, and research involving human embryos to eligibility for these services, payment to donors and surrogates, and on and on. Only portions of these statements are relevant to our concerns, but I thought I'd share with you a few brief highlights.

"Very quickly, then, on this topic: fifteen different committees from eight countries (Australia, the United Kingdom, the United States, Canada, the Federal Republic of Germany, France, the Netherlands, and Spain) issued extended statements. All fifteen held that IVF is acceptable in principle. Those that discussed the freezing of embryos all approved it, as well as their disposal. However, on the question of whether human embryo research is acceptable in principle, four of the fifteen committees said no. It's interesting to note that three of those four were different committees convened in Australia to study these issues. Of the eighty-five committees I mentioned earlier, nineteen were Australian."

"Bill, what was the other country that rejected embryo research in principle?"

"Let me see—oh, Tasmania."

"Really!"

"Where's Tasmania?"

"It's an island in the South Pacific."

"Why do you suppose Tasmania is interested in in vitro fertilization and research on embryos?"

"Probably because it's near Australia."

"Okay, let's get back on track. All the committees that did accept human embryo research set a time limit: fourteen days in every case except the National Ethics Committee in France, which limited the duration of research to seven days. That's all I'll say for the moment about these international committees except to note that most of the recommendations issued by them do not have the force of law. As is true of committees and commissions in our country—including the task force we're all serving on here—their recommendations are rarely binding. But they are usually respected and often become incorporated in statutes enacted by legislatures.

"Even though I'm a lawyer, I think sometimes the attempt to codify recommendations goes too far. Take, for example, the Warnock Commission in England. Its report, issued back in July 1984, contained sixty-three recommendations, twenty-three of which proposed new British laws, including recommendations to create seven new crimes involving human reproduction and embryo research. One legal authority referred to that approach as 'legal overkill,' because it seemed premature to outlaw as criminal so many features of artificial reproduction.[27] For our purposes, I think it's best to concentrate on what's been happening in the United States.

"As you know, laws can be made by legislatures, in the form of statutes, and also by courts, which establish the common law. To date, there has been more activity by courts than by legislatures, but that's not surprising. When disputes arise, our way of settling them in this country is to run to court; that's what keeps us lawyers in business. One of the first cases I came across goes back to 1978. In that case a doctor, who objected to a couple's attempt to use IVF before obtaining an IRB review destroyed their incubating embryo—"

"Excuse me, Bill. What's an IRB?"

"Oh, sorry. It stands for institutional review board, the name for hospital and medical school committees that review human subjects research."

"Are these IRBs required to review in vitro fertilization procedures?"

"Strictly speaking, no, unless the procedures are done as part of a research protocol. As a matter of fact, there's been a good deal of debate over whether IVF *should* have been required to undergo IRB approval from the very beginning, since it was obviously an experimental procedure. However, it was introduced as a therapeutic procedure—a treatment for infertility—despite the fact that it was a highly innovative treatment. This doesn't mean there's been no scientific research on IVF; it only means that the procedure was not officially classified as research, which would have meant more scrutiny by such committees as IRBs. But even then, federal regulations governing research require only research sponsored by the National Institutes of Health to be reviewed by an IRB. Since the NIH has not been sponsoring in vitro fertilization, the facilities performing clinical IVF wouldn't have been legally required to have IRB review anyway.

"Let me pick up the thread again. In the 1978 case, which occurred at Columbia Presbyterian Hospital (an affiliate of Columbia University's

College of Physicians and Surgeons), the doctor destroyed the incubating embryos of a couple, and the couple sued. The jury awarded them $50,000 in damages for intentional infliction of emotional distress. The ruling implicitly recognized the couple's ownership of their embryos.[28]

"A more recent case that received lots of publicity was *Davis v. Davis*, first dealt with in 1989 by a trial court judge in Tennessee.[29] Junior L. Davis and his wife, Mary Sue, decided to divorce after nine years of marriage. The couple had undergone six attempts at IVF, then decided to try adoption; when that failed, they returned again to IVF. In their seventh attempt, two embryos were transferred to Mary Sue's womb and seven additional embryos were frozen for possible future use. The two implanted embryos failed to develop. When the couple decided to divorce, they disagreed about the fate of their frozen embryos. Mary Sue wanted to keep them for possible implantation; Junior sought veto power over her decision. Unable to resolve their dispute, they went to court for a resolution. Ethical and legal opinion was sharply divided on the question of which member of this couple should have control of the embryos. Perhaps equally unclear was the question of what considerations should determine the fate of such embryos.

"The judge, however, framed the central issue in terms not of who should get control but of whether the embryos were people or products. Relying exclusively on the testimony of one witness, Jerome Lejeune, a French right-to-life physician, the judge concluded that the seven frozen embryos 'are human beings . . . not property' and that 'human life begins at the moment of conception.' He ruled: 'It is to the manifest best interest of the children, in vitro, that they be made available for implantation to assure their opportunity for live birth; implantation is their sole and only hope for survival.' Now many commentators believe that the embryos were properly awarded to Mary Sue Davis, rather than to Junior Davis. But as in any ethical or legal argument, it is the reasons given that justify the conclusion. In my view, the judge in the Davis case came to the right conclusions but for the wrong reason.

"One way to think about how to decide a dispute like this, where there's been no prior agreement between the two persons involved, is to ask, who would be harmed most by a ruling that favored the other party? It's my view that Mary Sue Davis would be harmed more than her husband, since these embryos may have represented her last chance to achieve a pregnancy. At the time the dispute arose, she was already thirty-seven. The biological clock was ticking. If this could really be her last shot at pregnancy, I think she'd be harmed more by giving her husband veto power over her decision to implant the embryos than he would be by being denied that power. A separate argument that would also favor the woman in such cases is referred to as the 'sweat equity' position—the woman has put more effort into production of the embryo, having undergone ovarian stimulation and surgical retrieval of her eggs.[30]

"Not everyone agrees with my view, though. John Robertson, a specialist in reproductive law, proposed an analysis resolving the case in favor of Junior Davis. Robertson argued that as a father, Junior would suffer significant financial and psychosocial burdens if unwanted reproduction occurred. This analysis did recognize a competing burden on the woman who fails to have the embryos available for transfer: 'Since one person's loss is the other person's gain, it may appear that there is no objective way to arbitrate the dispute.' Nevertheless, Robertson concluded, 'the party who wishes to avoid offspring is irreversibly harmed if embryo transfer and birth occur, for the burdens of unwanted parenthood cannot then be avoided,' whereas the woman, though frustrated by her inability to transfer these embryos, could still reproduce at a later time with other embryos.[31]

"Eight months after Mary Sue Davis won custody of the seven embryos, she opted to donate them to a fertility clinic so they could be used by another childless couple. She had remarried in the interim and declined to disclose her reason for changing her mind. Her former husband appealed the original court ruling. He was quoted as saying: 'There is just no way I am going to donate them. I feel that's my right. If there was a child from them, then I would be a parent to it. And I don't want a child out there to be mine if I can't be a parent to it.'[32] Whatever we may have thought of Junior Davis's claim to the embryos when his divorced wife wanted to have them implanted in herself, it's another story entirely if she decides to give them away. I said earlier that I was on the side of Mary Sue when she was seeking what might have been her last chance to achieve a pregnancy. But that basis for awarding her the embryos was no longer applicable, once she offered to donate them to another couple. At that point, the burden to Junior Davis became the only morally relevant consideration, since there was no longer any compensating benefit to his former wife.

"In 1990 the Tennessee Court of Appeals reversed the lower court's decision, giving the parties 'joint control' and an equal voice in the embyros' disposition. The court cited Mr. Davis's constitutional right to privacy, protecting his choice not to father a child; it found no compelling state interest in ordering implantatation against the will of one of the parties.[33]

The case eventually reached the Tennessee Supreme Court, which affirmed the appellate court's ruling but on somewhat different grounds. Following the analysis given by Robertson, the legal scholar I referred to earlier, the Tennessee Supreme Court said: 'The issue centers on the two aspects of procreational autonomy—the right to procreate and the right to avoid procreation.' In this case and similar ones, 'the party wishing to avoid procreation should prevail, assuming that the other party has a reasonable possibility of achieving parenthood by means other than the use of the pre-embryos in question.'[34] The practical result of this ruling is most likely to favor the party who objects, since there must be no other reasonable means available in order for the one seeking to become a parent to prevail.

"Another case, at about the same time the Davis case first came to court, also involved a dispute over frozen embryos. In *Jones v. York*, a couple who had been using the services of an IVF program in Virginia moved to California and wanted to transport their remaining frozen embryo to a Los Angeles clinic. The Norfolk, Virginia, program's refusal to grant them permission was based on a consent form they had signed, the fact that an institutional review board had not approved the transfer, and the risks of legal liability. Curiously, the Norfolk clinic also cited 'the demeaning effect' of shipping human embryos by air like 'cattle embryos.'[35] That's beginning to sound a bit like the judge in the Davis case, who held that the seven frozen embryos were 'human beings existing as embryos,' and 'children in vitro' whose best interests required 'that they be available for implantation.'[36]

"The court in the Virginia case, however, denied the clinic's efforts to dismiss the lawsuit in which the couple tried to gain control of the embryo. The court relied on a technical legal provision known as a 'bailor-bailee relationship,' using the cryopreservation agreement as a basis for the obligation of the 'bailee' (the clinic) to return the embryo to the couple. The significance of this ruling is its assumption that embryos are the 'property' of the couple that supplies the gametes for in vitro fertilization when the contesting party is an IVF clinic or cryopreservation facility. It would be an entirely different matter, though, to treat frozen embryos as 'property' if the contesting parties were competing parents, because preembryos 'cannot be divided to reflect partial "ownership." Once combined, the genetic material donated by each "owner" cannot be retrieved.'[37]

"Although there's much more to be said about the legal status of pre-embryos and frozen preembryos, let me conclude with a few words about embryo research. This is a very muddy topic in state laws. At least twenty states have enacted laws that restrict fetal research, but these statutes are so vaguely worded that they would apply to embryo research, as well. Federal regulations are clearer on that point, since they define the fetus as 'the entity that exists from the time of implantation, thus exempting preimplantation embryos from their reach.' But up to now, the federal government has not funded either embryo or fetal research.[38] In this realm, as in almost every other area where new medical technologies are being applied to human reproduction, there is an array of constantly developing law."

"Thank you very much, Bill. With all you've told us, I'm sure it's still only the tip of the iceberg, so to speak. The floor is open for general discussion."

Teddi Chernacoff speaks without being recognized by the chair. "You may be interested to know that Mary Sue Davis is still battling for those embryos, even after the Tennessee Supreme Court decision. She and her lawyer were guests on the Sally Jessy Raphael show, along with Junior Davis's lawyer, and she kept referring to the embryos as 'my children.' She said her 'children' had a right to live, or words to that effect."

"Teddi, is that what you do during the workday, watch Sally Jessy Raphael?" Bill Ackerman inquires.

"Actually, no," Chernacoff replies. "I've never seen the show. I was a guest on this one, along with Mary Sue and the two lawyers."[39]

"Is she still trying to donate them to another couple?"

"That wasn't entirely clear. She came through as wanting the embryos for herself but wasn't precise about it."

"I'm surprised you consented to be on the show," Andrea Goldwoman muses.

Chernacoff is about to defend herself when Tod Nielsen interrupts: "I guess you didn't see the article in the paper just the other day. The gynecologist who was storing the embryos turned them over to Junior Davis. Mr. Davis then disposed of them, but neither he nor his lawyer would comment on how the embryos were destroyed."[40]

The task force members begin buzzing until Maura O'Brien intervenes: "Any questions for Bill Ackerman?"

Roberta Bernstein raises her hand. "I have a question about the time period allowed for embryo research. Bill, you said these different international committee statements all set an outer limit of two weeks, and one statement put the limit at seven days. Why is that? After all, if a woman can abort a fetus any time within the first trimester, and maybe even up to the time of viability, why this restriction on embryo research? Isn't it inconsistent? Wouldn't it be more ethically consistent to treat all unborn life in a similar manner, setting the same limits on the age of an embryo and a fetus for purposes of what may be done to it?"

Bill Ackerman demurs. "Well, you know, these are just committee statements. They don't have the force of law."

"That doesn't really answer the question, Bill," Teddi Chernacoff chimes in. "I think we have to look at just what the purpose is, and who's making the decision, before we can conclude that ethical consistency requires that we treat all these entities in the same manner."

"We also have to look at whether these 'entities,' as you call them, are inside a woman's body or in a glass dish or a freezer," Andrea Goldwoman adds.

"I agree," Chernacoff continues. "It's important to note that a different relationship exists with the embryo or fetus in each of these cases. The researcher views an embryo as a means to the end of conducting biomedical research and has no other interest in it. But a woman with an unwanted pregnancy, or one carrying a fetus discovered to have a genetic defect, stands in an entirely different relationship to the fetus."

"I must insist that those are not morally relevant considerations," Father Reardon remarks. "At the risk of sounding like a broken record, I have to say once again that the centrality of human dignity at all stages of life demands that we respect the human embryo. This doesn't lead to a prohibition of any or all research on embryos. Under certain limited conditions, living embryos may be the subjects of experimentation, but the only valid reason is a therapeutic one: that is, when experimental therapy may provide some benefit to the embryo itself. Since the embryo or fetus cannot decide whether to participate in research, experiments for the benefit of society alone would be ruled out. Also ruled out, for certain, is the idea of keeping embryos alive for the sake of experimentation." [41]

"For those of us whose religion does not prohibit using embryos in these ways," Bernstein says, "I'm still waiting to hear an answer to my concern about consistency."

Chernacoff tries again. "A researcher is using an embryo solely as a means to an end. Yet even when a woman decides to have an abortion, and thus to terminate fetal life, she still has a relationship with her fetus. Very few women take a decision to abort lightly."

"But isn't the fetus still being used as a means? As a means to the woman's chosen ends? What's the difference whether it's a researcher's ends or a woman's ends for which an embryo or fetus is being used as a means?" Vera Rodriguez asks.

"I can only repeat the point," Chernacoff replies. "A woman stands in a different relationship to her fetus than a researcher does to an embryo."

"That answer still doesn't make it clear why the difference is a morally relevant one," Tod Nielsen remarks. "You're always instructing us on the need for justification, Teddi. Now I think you've failed to provide one."

"It's the best I can do at the moment."

"Any other questions?" Maura O'Brien surveys the group.

LeRoy Johnson raises his hand. "I'd just like to say, for the record, that we should try to keep these discussions separate and distinct from the abortion debate. I thought we had settled that in this state, in favor of the right of a woman to control her reproductive life. Our charge on this commission is to look at new reproductive technologies, and I think we should stick to that."

"Right on!" Goldwoman sings out.

Maura O'Brien looks at her watch. "It's now ten past ten, and some members of the task force have more than an hour's drive to get home. I'm going to close the meeting now, and remind you that next month we'll begin our discussion of surrogacy. The staff will be in touch about detailed arrangements, and we'll ask a few of you to make brief oral presentations as we did this evening. Meeting adjourned. Have a safe trip home."

❀

Larry and Bonnie rise as the task force members gather up their papers. "Larry, that's the bioethicist we consulted about the ethics of using artificial means of reproduction. Do you think she'd remember us?"

"Who knows? What difference does it make?"

"Well, I'd just like to say hello to her. Do you mind?"

"Why should I mind? Be my guest."

Bonnie edges over to where Chernacoff stands talking to other committee members and waits. When the group breaks up, Bonnie ventures timidly:

"Hi, Professor Chernacoff, I don't know if you remember me. My name's Bonnie Roberts. My husband and I talked to you last month about our own problem. I just wanted to thank you. It was very helpful."

"I'm glad to hear that. Of course I remember you. What did you decide to do?"

"We haven't quite decided. That's why we came here tonight."

"You're welcome to attend any time. These are open meetings. The committee has nothing to hide, and we believe our deliberations should be available to all citizens, as well as to the press."

"Thanks again."

Larry and Bonnie walk out silently. "That was interesting," Bonnie remarks.

"It didn't help us any," Larry replies.

"I still think it was interesting. Why don't we come again next month when they discuss surrogacy?"

"We'll see."

Conflicting Views about Surrogacy

Bonnie fidgets while Larry watches the football game. Eventually she complains, "If we don't make some sort of decision soon, I'll go crazy. Can't we talk soon—now—about what we're going to do?"

"Okay, I promise. As soon as the game is over, I'll give you my undivided attention."

Bonnie has assembled a large manila envelope full of clippings about the Baby M case. She has studied the clippings so that she'll have answers to anything Larry might ask. Before she broaches the subject of surrogacy, she wants to make sure he has no objections to other features of the new reproductive technologies.

"What did you really think about the discussion we heard at the task force meeting?"

"I already told you what I thought. It didn't have much to do with us."

"Yes it did, in a way. I mean, I came away with the idea that there's probably nothing immoral about using these artificial means of reproduction."

"Yeah, I guess so."

"You don't agree with the arguments of the Catholic priest, do you Larry?"

"I'm not Catholic. Why do you even ask?"

"Some people who aren't Catholic agree with those arguments. Just look at this article I xeroxed in the library. It's called 'The Ethics of Human Manufacture,' and it talks about 'artificial babies,' 'artificial families,' and 'artificial sex.'[1] And it appeared in a very liberal magazine, the *New Republic*."

"What's it say?"

"Well, for one thing, the author says that test-tube babies, synthetic families, and synthetic sex all pose moral problems."[2]

"What, for example?"

"I'll read a section or two. Here, the author says: 'The inner core of the Church's concern about the new reproductive science is—correctly, in my view—the new technologies of fetal manipulation that are drifting into legitimation. . . . moral dilemmas posed by the new reproductive technology [include] threats to the dignity of the individual, to the integrity of the family, and to the "unity" (perhaps ultimately to the utility) of sex.' "[3]

"I'm sorry, Bonnie, I don't understand what all that means. What's his real point?"

"I confess, I don't exactly know. He thinks the church has a right to make such declarations, but the liberal state doesn't have that right. But he ends the article by saying we have to 'avoid the horrors of the new reproductive science.' "[4]

Larry takes the photocopy from Bonnie and skims it. "Well, maybe I'm dense, but it doesn't make sense to me."

"At this point, we know our only hope of having a child that's really ours is to use a surrogate mother. But before we can even think about that, we have to agree that there's nothing actually wrong with in vitro fertilization and the rest of what we'll have to go through. Including possibly throwing out or freezing some unused embryos."

"Nothing wrong with any of those things as far as I'm concerned. Now what are the problems with using a surrogate mother?"

"The main problem is, what if she decides she wants to keep the baby, like Mary Beth Whitehead did?"

"Oh, God help us! The last thing I need is to start going to court, hiring lawyers, having newspaper and TV reporters after us. Is that what we're letting ourselves in for?"

"Not necessarily. Only a few surrogates have actually tried to get their babies back. I read that others were unhappy about the arrangement, though. I don't know. That's why I think we should go back to the task force meeting next month when they discuss surrogacy."

"Okay, we'll go. But what else do we have to worry about?"

"The law, I guess. I read that some states have already passed laws that prohibit surrogacy for money. Michigan made it a crime."

"No kidding. A crime? You mean we could be criminals if we did this? Great!"

"Other states did just the opposite. They made surrogacy contracts legitimate—even commercial ones."

"I guess we'd better find out just what the law is."

"I still worry that a surrogate might want to keep the baby. But I don't think our situation would be like the Baby M case. Mary Beth Whitehead was artificially inseminated with William Stern's sperm, so the baby was really half hers. With us, it would be my egg and your sperm, so the surrogate mother wouldn't be the baby's biological mother. That makes a difference."

"I'm convinced. But what would a judge say, if it ever comes to that?"

"I don't know. But now I'm going to find out what our surrogacy options are."

❀

Knowing that the Fecundity Center's reproductive services include a matching program for couples and surrogates, Bonnie calls for more information and learns that the clinic will either arrange for the services of a surrogate through a broker, for a fee, or else perform the procedure with a surrogate of the couple's own choosing. In the latter case, there would not need to be an additional fee paid to the surrogate, but the clinic would still be paid for medical and psychiatric screening and for doing the egg retrieval, in vitro fertilization, and subsequent embryo transfer.

Larry and Bonnie still want to make certain that what they now plan to do is legal. Although they have no reason to suspect that the Fecundity

Center is operating outside the law, they decide to consult an attorney. First they call the lawyer they used when they bought their house. When they tell him the nature of the legal advice they are seeking, he is stumped.

"I don't know a thing about that stuff. I just do ordinary commercial law, divorces, real estate, and that sort of thing. This is a very specialized area."

"Yeah," Larry acknowledges, "but you must know more than we do."

"Not necessarily," the lawyer replies. "But I'll ask around in my firm and see if anyone can help."

When the attorney calls back in two days, he has only disappointing news. "Larry, no one here knows anything about reproductive laws."

"Can't you ask someone in another law firm? Or in another city? There must be someone in New York or L.A. who knows something."

"Okay, I'll give it another try. But if this search begins to take up too much time, I'll have to start billing you."

The lawyer calls the state bar association and is referred to the American Bar Association, family law section. He is given the name of Warren Blackstein, a law professor with expertise in this area. The lawyer transmits the name to Larry and Bonnie and wishes them luck.

Bonnie calls Blackstein's office and makes an appointment for the following week. When they arrive for their consultation, the professor ushers them into his law school office. "Welcome. I understand you're looking for information about the law in this state regarding surrogacy. Well, the bad news is, at present there is no law. And from your point of view, the good news is the same: at present there is no law."

"Where does that leave us?" Bonnie asks.

"I can outline for you what the possibilities are, but that's all. Two bills have been introduced into the state legislature, and it's anybody's guess what will happen. The bills are quite different. Also keep in mind that in our tri-state area one neighboring state has proposed legislation and the other has already passed a law. There's been a flurry of activity everywhere; since 1980, legislation related to surrogate motherhood has been introduced in over half the state legislatures.[5] During the 1987 legislative sessions alone, approximately seventy-two surrogacy bills were introduced in twenty-six states and the District of Columbia.[6] It's amazing how these bills differ. Some would permit and regulate surrogacy contracts, while others would prohibit these arrangements entirely or partially, or make them unenforceable by a court.[7] At this point, sixteen states have passed laws regarding surrogacy. But I must tell you, most of these statutes deal with only some of the many issues raised by surrogacy."

Bonnie ventures, "But I read that somewhere—Michigan, I think—surrogacy was criminalized."

"Right, commercial surrogacy arrangements have been made criminal offenses in Michigan. But that doesn't concern us—although, to be honest, one of the bills introduced in our state is virtually identical to the Michigan law."

"Aaargh!" Larry groans. "Is this really a good idea, then?"

"Let me tell you about the features of these different bills, and then you can decide."

Professor Blackstein begins by outlining features of the first act proposed in their state.[8] According to this proposal, surrogacy agreements (including commercial arrangements) would be valid once approved by a court of appropriate jurisdiction. In the absence of judicial approval, however, such agreements would be null and void. The bill refers to the surrogate as a "surrogate mother."[9] It states that after carrying the child to term, she shall "relinquish the custody of the child conceived to the intended parents immediately after the child's birth or as soon thereafter as medically feasible."[10] The bill provides for "just and reasonable monetary compensation for the surrogate mother," but it prohibits contractual provisions "whereby compensation is conditioned upon the health, viability, or survival of the child at term."[11] Professor Blackstein concludes his description of the bill by quoting the following provision: "Any child born to a surrogate mother shall be deemed the legitimate, natural child of the intended parents for all purposes."

Blackstein cautions: "This is the more favorable bill of the two introduced into the state legislature. The second proposal would prohibit all paid surrogacy arrangements but would allow agreements in which the surrogate mother is unpaid."[12]

The professor outlines the features of this second bill, pointing out its similarity to provisions in the law governing adoption. Like the Michigan statute, the bill would prohibit commercial surrogacy and attach criminal penalties to violators. Also prohibited would be payments to agents and intermediaries—including attorneys and physicians—as finders' fees for locating volunteer mothers or for matching a volunteer mother with an intended couple. Noncommercial surrogacy would not be prohibited but would be strictly regulated. For example, the "volunteer mother" (as the surrogate is called in this bill) must agree to become pregnant by the fertility method specified in a prior adoption agreement. The surrogate would terminate her parental rights to the child she bears through a written consent executed at the time the adoption agreement is signed. However, the surrogate would have a right to rescind this contract at any time within seven days of the birth of the child.

"You mean, the law would actually support the right of the surrogate to keep the baby?" Bonnie is incredulous.

"Yes, in the same way adoption law does. A pregnant woman who decides during pregnancy to give her baby up for adoption still has a legal right to change her mind within a specified period of time after the birth of the child."

"That makes it kind of risky, doesn't it?" Larry asks.

"That's true, once a law like this is in effect. But remember, not all women who enter these sorts of arrangements end up wanting to keep the baby. The vast majority do not."

"But how can we tell in advance? It seems to me that just asking the surrogate mother isn't very good insurance."

"There are no guarantees under such laws. You're right, you just have to take your chances."

Bonnie is on the verge of tears.

"Look, Bon, don't get all worked up just yet. Professor Blackstein said these are just proposed laws; they haven't been passed yet. Maybe if we work quick enough, we can get it all done before the legislature acts."

Blackstein reminds Larry, "You wouldn't be absolutely safe in any event. Remember the Baby M case. Even without a statute, a surrogate would still have recourse to the courts. Would you like me to describe briefly the law already passed in our neighboring state? Just for the sake of completeness?"

"Sure, why not?"

"You're not going to like this one."

Professor Blackstein proceeds to outline a statute that assigns criminal penalties to commercial surrogacy arrangements and is discouraging to noncommercial surrogacy arrangements as well.[13] This law makes it a felony for persons other than participating parties to induce, arrange, procure, or otherwise assist in the formation of a surrogate parentage contract for compensation. The penalty is a fine of not more than $50,000 or imprisonment for not more than five years, or both. Participating parties who knowingly enter into a surrogate parentage contract for compensation are guilty of a misdemeanor punishable by a fine of not more than $10,000 or imprisonment for not more than five years, or both. "Participating parties" are defined as the biological mother or father and the surrogate carrier, and the spouse of a biological mother, father, or surrogate carrier. If a child is born of a surrogacy arrangement and there is a dispute between the parties concerning custody, the party having physical custody of the child may retain physical custody until the circuit court orders otherwise. The court's determination shall be based on "the best interests of the child."[14]

"We're definitely not going to that state!" Larry grunts.

"That's about all I can tell you regarding the present legal situation now," Blackstein concludes. "If you have any more questions, I'll be glad to try to answer them."

Bonnie and Larry are silent as they drive home. "It's worth a try," Larry muses.

"I agree. But first, let's hear what the Reproductive Task Force has to say. We've already decided to go to the meeting, so we can make up our minds after hearing arguments pro and con."

❖

At 6:40 P.M. Maura O'Brien calls the task force meeting to order. "We have a full agenda this evening, so let's get started. We've scheduled several brief presentations of the various and opposing points of view on surrogacy as background for our discussion. Some readings were distributed in advance, and I hope you all received them. We mailed everyone a complete copy of the New Jersey Supreme Court decision in the Baby M case. The first presentation will be by Tod Nielsen. Tod?"

"Maura asked me to give an account of surrogacy arrangements based on the notion of reproductive freedom. She also asked me to defend the idea of commercial surrogacy. I'm not sure I really believe everything I'm about to say, but I'm trying to do a service by making the most convincing case I can. So here goes.

"An argument can be made that an individual's or couple's right to 'procreative autonomy' includes the right to contract with consenting adults for the purpose of bearing a child. Another right, the right to 'genetic continuity,' can be cited as part of the right of reproductive choice.[15] Substantial civil liberties interests are at issue here, interests that should be respected as a matter of law, including constitutional law. Constitutional rights include the right to privacy and autonomy in an array of intimate sexual, social, and family relationships involving bodily integrity, personal choice, and future association with offspring.[16] The constitutional protections regarding privacy are well known in the areas of contraception and abortion.

Perhaps less well known is the fact that the Supreme Court has held that natural parents have a constitutionally protected interest in the rearing of their child.[17]

"Extending these rights into the arena of surrogacy, I can identify a number of rights and interests that support the legal validity of surrogacy arrangements. First there are the private relationships and procreative intentions of the various parties. Then there is the right of a woman (the surrogate, I mean) to control her own body. Next there are the rights of biological parents to associate with their child. The biological father, who usually initiates the whole process, has an emotional commitment and deep desire to have a genetically related child. This entitles him to be treated as a parent and to claim a privacy right consistent with that status.[18]

"A common objection raised against surrogacy is the commercial aspect. Yet it can be argued that that aspect, too, should be legally permitted.[19] There are numerous examples of commercial arrangements in parenting: paying sperm donors in connection with artificial insemination, paying women who donate their eggs, the costs of carrying out adoption procedures, and others. Surrogacy should be no different. One argument against permitting payment to a surrogate comes out in the analogy with adoption. It is true that treating a child as a commodity is unconstitutional and contrary to public policy: baby-selling is a crime in most jurisdictions, and some people claim that surrogacy contracts are very similar to paid adoption.[20] But it is questionable whether payment to a surrogate should be construed as a form of baby-selling. It is more plausibly viewed as remuneration for the surrogate's services for a nine-month period of time.

"Moreover, there is ample reason to reject the analogy with adoption. Adoption involves an unwanted child, while surrogacy is premised on a very much wanted child. This is why some of the features common to adoption practices should not apply to surrogacy. What I have in mind here is mainly the surrender of the infant following birth. The surrogacy agreement is a contract, and the terms of a contract should be fulfilled, morally and legally. On the analogy with adoption, some states have required a waiting period after the birth of the child before the surrogate turns over the baby to the intended rearing parents. There should be no waiting period. This view is common among many professionals; at the trial after Mary Beth Whitehead refused to relinquish Baby M, a physician testified that she was simply a 'surrogate uterus.'[21] And in at least one state, Arkansas, the law clearly provides that the intended parents are the legal parents.[22]

"If surrogates weren't paid for their reproductive services, the practice of surrogacy would dry up quickly. Who would enter such an arrangement without being paid? To quote Noel Keane, the lawyer from Michigan who has been arranging surrogate contracts for fifteen years, 'Unless surrogate mothers can be offered meaningful compensation for their services, very few children will be brought legally into the world in this manner.'[23] The end of the practice of surrogacy would be a cause for great unhappiness on the part of many infertile couples. Besides, I suspect that if payments were legally prohibited, money would flow under the table. The result would be clandestine behavior and the creation of a new class of 'criminals'—parties to a paid surrogacy agreement.

"Surrogacy will continue, whether it is banned, outlawed, or subjected to civil or criminal penalties. It stems from deeply rooted human feelings— the desire for a child who is biologically related to at least one parent. Since surrogate parenting cannot be legislated out of existence, therefore, the best option is to regulate it in order to prevent abuses. This task force could choose an approach in a range of options from criminal prohibition at one end of a continuum to encouraging surrogacy at the other end. I think a decision to have a child by using a surrogate is an intensely private one and should remain so in a free society. The state has no business interfering in people's reproductive lives. I think the state should remain neutral about the substance of surrogacy, acting only in a regulatory capacity. Statutory limits could be set on payments to surrogates, and other provisions should be included in legislation to protect the parties from being harmed or wronged. If carefully regulated to prevent abuses, surrogacy can become just another social option for citizens to choose freely."

Seven hands shoot up as Tod Nielsen finishes.

"Are these questions of information, or substantive comments?" Maura O'Brien asks.

"Tod, what if a defective child is born of a surrogacy arrangement?"

"Does the contracting couple have a right to control the surrogate mother's behavior during pregnancy?"

"What if the surrogate has medical problems as a result of pregnancy or childbirth? What follows then?"

"What about physical and mental screening for surrogates? What are the standards here?"

"What is likely to be the impact on children born of these arrangements? Don't they stand to be harmed?"

Maura interrupts. "I'm going to rule all these questions out of order at the moment. They are all relevant and important, but they go beyond the topic Tod was asked to address. I'd like to go on with the other brief presentations now. Remember, some of the questions just posed are the issues we'll be grappling with on this task force in the months to come. Could we hear next from Father Reardon, please."

"Thank you, Ms. O'Brien. The last time I addressed this group I presented the views of the Roman Catholic church on artificial modes of reproduction. Of course, to the extent that surrogate motherhood involves the use of these artificial modes of reproduction, it is illicit because *they* are illicit, according to church teaching. But there are additional considerations that militate against surrogacy, considerations so weighty that many people who accept other artificial forms of reproduction are nonetheless adamantly opposed to surrogacy. Some of these considerations have been articulated in secular law: for example, in the decision handed down by the New Jersey Supreme Court in the matter of Baby M. I'll be referring to that judicial decision at various points in my presentation. But I want mainly to focus on some of the religious concerns about surrogate motherhood.[24]

"Children are a gift of God. As such they can never be treated as chattels or commercial pawns or as commodities to be produced in exchange for a fee. As the New Jersey Supreme Court so cogently said: 'There are, in a civilized society, some things that money cannot buy.' The practice of surrogate motherhood is an affront to the human dignity of a child. The whole activity reduces the creation of a child, a human being, to the level of a commercial transaction. The womb is leased to produce rather than to love a child into existence. When the natural mother relinquishes her child for pay, she is exploiting the most precious thing she can bring into existence. In surrogacy, unlike adoption, a child is conceived precisely in order to be abandoned to others, and his or her best interests are the last factors to be considered.

"We must also take heed of the rights of the child. Every child has a right to true parents. Surrogacy confounds the relationship by introducing a second mother. This results in a denial of the natural attachment a woman has to the child in whose creation she has participated. Further, it destroys the parent-child bond, and the child suffers a grave injustice. A great potential exists for psychological injury to a child who learns that he or she was born from a cold, usually financial relationship rather than a loving relationship.

"Surrogacy also involves the exploitation of women as part of a 'human machine.' After the surrogate mother uses her womb for a commercial purpose, her work is accomplished, her contract labor finished, and she is made to surrender an integral part of her life, her child, and with it any natural claim or bond to that child. To terminate the mother's rights simply fails to take account of the natural bonding between mother and child. A related problem is the likelihood of exploitation of poor women. Undue pressure may lead poor women to use their bodies in this manner to support themselves or their families. Is this not a new form of prostitution?

"The opposition to surrogate motherhood on the part of the church I represent is broader than laws against commercial surrogacy. We favor banning not only commercial surrogacy but all surrogacy arrangements whatsoever. Whether commercial or voluntary, surrogate motherhood is morally wrong because it violates the biological and spiritual unity of the husband and wife and the dignity of the person of the child who is made an object for which the parties negotiate. Sound social policy mandates the enactment of laws that uphold marriage and the family, long-cherished institutions. Marriage is a unitive covenant. To introduce a surrogate mother into the marital relationship to take on the procreative role is to undermine the unity of the relationship.

"The family is undermined in still other ways. Rather than a bond between husband and wife, a child born of a surrogate mother can readily become a divisive force. How does a surrogate's husband feel about having his wife's womb rented out? How are the surrogate's other children likely to feel, knowing that their mother sold or gave away their brother or sister? We must consider the rights, feelings, and interests of all the children who might be affected by such arrangements.

"Surrogate motherhood subverts the laws of nature. Who indeed should be considered the child's parent? The man whose sperm artificially inseminated the woman? The woman who produced the egg? Or the woman who carried the child and gave it birth?

"In sum, then, surrogacy promotes the exploitation of women and infertile couples and the dehumanization of babies. Commercial surrogacy traffics for profit in human lives. A society that has overturned the institution of slavery and, moreover, does not allow the sale of human organs should certainly not allow the sale of a child. The practice of voluntary surrogacy is equally repugnant, as it is wholly incompatible with the sanctity of marriage and the nurturing of the family. I hope this task force will see fit to recommend legal prohibition of all forms of surrogacy."

Maura O'Brien nods at Andrea Goldwoman, who prefaces her presentation with some explanatory remarks. "As you recall, last month I gave a feminist account of the new reproductive technologies. I had prepared at that time a section on surrogacy, which Maura asked me to reserve for tonight's meeting. You'll also recall that Teddi was critical of my feminist analysis of the new reproductive technologies, correctly pointing out that not all feminists speak with one voice. So I gave some thought to what I had prepared to say tonight, and made some revisions. I decided to separate out my own views, which tend to follow the more radical feminist line, and tell you something about the division within the feminist community on this issue. I realize I was appointed to this task force not merely to be an advocate for my own views and those of WARO but also to contribute more general information about feminist thinking on these issues.

"As an example of the feminist split on the issue of surrogacy, take the National Organization for Women. During the Baby M trial the New Jersey chapter of NOW held a meeting and failed to reach consensus. The head of the chapter was reported to have said: 'We do believe that women ought to control their own bodies, and we don't want to play big brother or big sister and tell them what to do. . . . But on the other hand, we don't want to see the day when women are turned into breeding machines.'[25]

"I'd also like to say a word about Father Reardon's presentation. Much of what Father had to say is heartily endorsed by feminists. This may come as some surprise, since on many issues feminists and the Roman Catholic church take opposing sides. There are exceptions, however, even in the most obvious area, the abortion controversy. There is a group that calls itself 'Catholics for Choice,' and another group known as 'Feminists for Life.' But on the issue of surrogacy, the position that Father Reardon presented is one that many feminists accept, and for some of the same reasons.

"Father Reardon wondered whether surrogacy isn't another, newer form of prostitution. Well, many feminists agree; they refer to the practice as 'reproductive prostitution.' On the other hand, as distasteful as prostitution is to many people, there are feminists who believe that the state has no right to prohibit a woman from selling the sexual use of her body.[26] So, if the state shouldn't interfere with a woman's choice to become a prostitute, why should it be able to prohibit her from selling the reproductive use of her body?

"It's clear, then, that feminists are divided on the issue of surrogacy, as radical feminists and the liberal wing are on the general issue of reproductive technologies—the split Teddi described at the last meeting. But when it comes to surrogacy, the liberal feminists are ambivalent. I think their ambivalence reflects the ambivalence of society as a whole on this topic. There is one point on which all feminists are united, though. That's the point about control of the surrogate's behavior during pregnancy. No feminist I've ever read or heard accepts the idea that the surrogate's behavior should be limited in any way, before or during the pregnancy, in accordance with provisions stated in a surrogacy contract.

"Since future meetings will be devoted to exploring the various stances on commercial surrogacy—who gets the baby in disputed surrogacy arrangements, whether surrogacy contracts should be made illegal or unenforceable, and the rest of the contested areas—I'll spend the remainder of my time here giving the essence of the radical feminist position. I will be brief.

"Radical feminists hold that surrogacy exploits women in general, as well as the particular women who 'choose' to act as surrogates. We believe that such women aren't really exercising free choice, that they don't really choose in a voluntary manner. There is always an element of coercion involved, even if coercion operates at a societal rather than a personal level. Surrogacy demeans all women, not just the women who enter into such arrangements. Since any practice that demeans at least half the population should be prohibited by law, we believe that surrogacy should be outlawed.

"Radical feminists reject the 'liberty line' propounded by civil libertarians and most of the liberal feminists. 'We hear lots of highminded talk about "rights" and "liberty" from the defenders of the human breeding industry. It's a man's right to exercise his constitutionally protected and newly invented "procreative liberty" to hire a woman to bear a child for him.'[27] Gary Skoloff, the lawyer for William Stern in the Baby M case, spouted the liberty line. You heard Tod Nielsen spouting the same line here earlier this evening, as do some of my feminist sisters from the liberal wing. And, of course, 'this liberty line has been eagerly grabbed by the surrogacy industry.' But this is 'junk liberty' and must be exposed for what it is. 'Human rights must be based on human dignity, and surrogacy, which violates human dignity, is no "right."'[28]

"Surrogacy involves the objectification, sale, and commodification of a woman's body. It is nothing other than reproductive prostitution and is therefore a crime against women. 'The crime is turning a whole class of people—women—into a commodity exchange, and in so doing, violating our human dignity.'[29] Systematic exploitation of any individuals or groups should be prohibited. So, radical feminists agree with the position of the Catholic church in holding that surrogacy is against public policy, a position I hope this task force will adopt. Thank you."

Maura O'Brien turns to the bioethicist. "Teddi, I hope you'll clear things up for us, in your usual lucid manner. Could you give us an ethical analysis of everything we've heard so far about surrogacy?"

"A tall order, but I'll try. Forgive me for getting a bit theoretical, but I think some background in ethical theory will be useful in helping to frame the debate over surrogacy.[30]

"A reasoned approach to the ethics of surrogacy can proceed by using either of two well-known ethical perspectives. The first examines the good and bad consequences of an action or practice as a means of determining its moral rightness or wrongness, while the second tries to determine whether an act or practice is inherently or intrinsically wrong.

"According to the first ethical perspective—consequentialism—if the good consequences outweigh the bad, the action or practice is ethically acceptable. If, on the other hand, there is a balance of bad consequences over good ones, then the action or practice is morally wrong. The method requires looking at alternative courses of action and their various possible outcomes, comparing the positive and negative features of those outcomes, and then determining which course of action has the most favorable balance of good consequences.

"Although the consequentialist approach is theoretically sound, it is fraught with many practical difficulties. Not only is it difficult to predict good and bad results; it's also hard to weigh consequences, even those that have already come about. Moreover, reasonable people frequently disagree over what should count as good and bad consequences, and how much weight should be assigned to each.

"It's worth noting that hundreds—maybe even thousands—of surrogacy arrangements have been successfully completed, with a distinct minority resulting in regrets by the surrogate mother, and only a few leading to the sorts of devastating consequences exemplified by the Baby M case. For example, figures from California show that only about one percent of the estimated five hundred surrogate birth arrangements made in that state during the past decade have ended in a legal dispute.[31] If applying the utilitarian principle were simply a matter of counting the individuals who experienced good consequences, those who experienced bad consequences, and subtracting, it would be an easy matter to determine the rightness or wrongness of surrogacy. But a proper application of the principle is methodologically much more complex. It requires assessing the magnitude of the good and bad consequences for every individual affected by the action or practice, a task abounding in problems of measurement and interpersonal comparisons.

"The competing approach to ethics rejects consequences as largely irrelevant. This approach holds that certain actions are wrong because of the very type of action they are. Some types of actions are intrinsically wrong. Examples include the killing of innocent human beings, the enslavement of individuals or groups, economic or social exploitation of persons or classes, and physical or mental torture. Of course, debates continue to rage over just which human beings should be considered 'innocent,' whether some living entities, such as fetuses, should be considered human beings, and just what should count as economic or social exploitation. But such debates do not detract from the respectability of this approach to ethics.

"In tackling the issue of surrogacy broadly, the first fundamental ethical question is whether there is something intrinsically wrong with surrogacy arrangements. Is this a practice whose very nature makes it immoral? Does surrogate motherhood violate some basic ethical principle? Those who believe it does argue that surrogacy ought to be outlawed, not simply regulated. They contend that the practice of surrogacy is morally flawed in principle, and that erecting safeguards cannot erase its fundamental ethical wrong. Within this category fall the objections of the Roman Catholic church and some feminist groups, as we've already heard this evening.

"While some critics of surrogate motherhood base their opposition on the interests of the children or on the motives of the surrogates, others are opposed because of what they claim is exploitation of women. This makes it appear that surrogacy is unethical because of the type of practice it is: namely, a form of exploitation. Both Father Reardon and Ms. Goldwoman criticized surrogacy on those grounds. According to one article in the literature, 'When a woman provides womb service, the feminist issue surfaces. Women object to being baby factories or sex objects because it offends their human dignity.'[32] This author, who is a feminist and a Catholic, makes an additional claim: 'This is going to end up as the final exploitation of women. It is always going to be poor women who have the babies and rich women who get them.'[33]

"These statements, however, confuse two distinct issues: first, the exploitation of individual women, if that is indeed what really happens in surrogacy arrangements; and second, a form of class exploitation, since poorer women will be the ones serving as surrogates for the more well-to-do. My own view is that these would be sound, principled objections if it were clear that exploitation in some form actually occurs.

"When feminists charge that the practice of surrogacy exploits women, they are being paternalistic. They are questioning women's ability to know their own interests and to enter a contractual arrangement knowingly and competently. There may well be a coercive aspect to commercial surrogacy, since money—especially a large enough sum—can serve as a coercive inducement to do something a person might not do voluntarily. But that speaks more to the exploitation of poorer classes of women, which I think is a genuine moral worry, than it does to the exploitation of women generally. Feminists who oppose surrogacy presume to speak for all women.

But what they are really saying is that those who elect to enter surrogacy arrangements are incompetent to choose and stand in need of protection.

"The charge of 'exploitation' contradicts the moral stance that women have the ability and the right to control their own bodies. If that right grants women reproductive freedoms of other sorts, such as the right to choose abortion or to control the number and spacing of their children, why does it not similarly apply to the informed, voluntary choice to serve as a surrogate? Radical feminists draw an analogy with prostitution, another practice believed to constitute exploitation of women. But the chief feminist complaint about prostitution pertains to its commercial aspect, the feature that transforms women's use of their bodies into a commodity. Feminists who see nothing wrong with women engaging in sexual intercourse outside of marriage (in today's terms—as long as they practice safer sex) are inconsistent if they contend that noncommercial surrogacy arrangements are demeaning to women.

"Still, it could be argued, to treat one's body as a mere means to the ends of others is degrading. It could be viewed as a violation of Kant's supreme moral principle, the categorical imperative, which prohibits treating persons merely as a means. But according to that interpretation, other acts and practices typically considered altruistic, even noble, might similarly have to be viewed as degrading. For instance, a normal, healthy volunteer of biomedical or behavioral research is also acting as a means to the ends of others—either of the researchers, or of future generations, or both. Of course, informed volunteers are not acting as a *mere* means, since their voluntary participation in research implies that they share or endorse the ends of scientific research. But what about the practice of paying research subjects for their participation? On the analogy with commercial surrogacy, such monetary payments would surely have to be outlawed, if it is exploitation to pay people for the use of their bodies or services that use their bodies.

"These analogies serve as a reminder that surrogate motherhood is a biomedical as well as a social practice, since it involves either artificial insemination or embryo transfer, then pregnancy and childbirth. It leads naturally to some considerations about informed consent.

"Although surrogacy arrangements are typically governed by a legal contract, the concept of informed consent is still applicable. Yet it has been argued that no one is capable of granting truly informed consent to be a surrogate mother. Most surrogacy arrangements require that women who offer to be surrogates already have children; this would seem to meet the objection that surrogate mothers cannot possibly know what it is like to go through pregnancy and childbirth. But those who claim that genuine informed consent is impossible contend that even if a woman has already borne children, she cannot know in advance what it is like to have to give up a child after birth.

"There is some merit to that contention. Yet as an argument against the very possibility of informed consent, it's too strong. If it holds for surrogate motherhood, it would seem to apply, as well, to a wide variety of other bio-medical treatments and research maneuvers that people have never before experienced. The only time patients could give truly informed consent to treatment would be in those cases where they have already undergone the same or very similar treatment. If the standard for gaining informed consent had to be interpreted in that way, it would lose much of its ordinary meaning. As an ethical and legal concept pertaining to medical therapy and research, informed consent requires that the person understand the likely consequences. It is unrealistic to maintain that the only way to gain such understanding is to have had the actual experience, along with the accompanying feelings.

"So, either the meaning of informed consent to become a surrogate mother is the same as that of informed consent to medical treatment, or it is different. If it should be understood in the usual sense, then a woman should be as capable of granting informed consent to carrying a baby to term and then relinquishing it as she is of granting consent to the removal of a breast when she has breast cancer, or removal of her uterus if she develops a tumor, or an operation to reduce or enlarge her breasts. If a different and higher standard of informed consent is to be used, however, then the only women who could qualify would be those who had already undergone the experience of having had a baby and lost it. But that would surely be a bizarre requirement, and probably a cruel one as well.

"A factor that complicates the debate at the policy level is the contention that surrogate motherhood is a form of baby-selling. When the attorney for Mary Beth Whitehead asserted that a contract to be a surrogate mother for money is 'against public policy,' he was referring to his belief that the contract violated state adoption laws and public policies against the sale of babies.

"Once again, this places the assessment of surrogacy in the context of a commercial arrangement. Although I have been urging that the commercial aspects be separated from the social arrangement of surrogacy for the purpose of ethical evaluation, the underlying conceptual question remains: is this a form of baby selling? Or should payment be considered more like a fee for services rendered? People who express a strong emotional distaste for surrogate motherhood are quick to label it baby-selling. That term has such negative connotations and the practice is so universally disapproved that once surrogacy is categorized as a new variety of baby-selling, its rejection is sure to follow quickly. But fairness demands an objective examination of the issue. It's an old trick of argumentation to apply a concept that already carries negative connotations to a different situation, with the aim of persuading listeners that the new situation should, like the old one, be viewed in a negative light. Philosophers call that 'persuasive definition.'

"A Kentucky court, holding that surrogate contracts do not violate public policy, asked how it is possible for a natural father to be accused of buying his own child.[34] My own view on this question is that paying a woman to be a surrogate mother is more like renting a womb than it is like buying a baby. Monetary payment is for the woman's inconvenience and possible discomfort, including the risks of any complications of pregnancy. This interpretation can be supported by looking at the features of surrogacy contracts, features that impose certain duties and obligations on the surrogate mother during pregnancy.

"Yet despite my conclusion that contracts for surrogacy should not be considered a form of baby-selling, and therefore in violation of laws that prohibit that activity, I believe it is morally wrong to undertake commercial surrogacy transactions. There are two arguments in support of this view.

"The first argument goes back to an earlier point: there is a risk that richer women will exploit those who are poorer or less advantaged. The magnitude of this danger is probably exaggerated by the opponents of surrogate motherhood. Yet it is surely true that women who are poor, uneducated, or both have fewer options than those who are better off financially. They are more likely to be unemployed, receiving welfare payments, or forced to remain at home caring for their own young children. For a woman in these circumstances the offer of money to bear the child of another woman is probably an undue inducement. It is an offer that may be difficult for a person of meager financial means to refuse and would, in that case, be coercive.

"Still, it would be hasty to conclude that any substantial amount of money offered to a person of small means, in return for services, is necessarily coercive. Payments to surrogates might be regulated so as to lessen the possibility of exploitation of the poor by the well-to-do. But what could serve as a proper basis for regulation? Although an offer of money is almost always an inducement to act in certain ways, it is difficult to determine when an incentive becomes an undue inducement.[35]

"One possibility would be to relativize payments to the financial status of the surrogate. With this maneuver, the problems posed by the other alternatives—leaving the entire matter to market forces, or seeking to devise a scheme of fixed payments—might be avoided. But a new difficulty would arise: to relativize acceptable monetary payments to each potential surrogate would result in providing different sums of money for essentially the same services. In effect, this would be giving unequal pay for equal work. Leaving aside the further complication that labor is much harder for some women than for others, nothing more need be said about the ethics of violating the precept of equal pay for equal work.

"There is a lingering worry. The presumption that wealthier women who seek to employ surrogates are exploiting them could be viewed as paternalistic, since it seems to imply that poor women may not be able to assess their own interests. Why shouldn't they be permitted to commit themselves for nine months to the obligations of carrying a pregnancy and get paid for their efforts?

"The answer to that question leads to considerations of justice. The particular concept of justice involved here is that of 'distributive justice.' Simply put, distributive justice requires that society's goods be distributed fairly among different social classes and racial and ethnic groups. Since it is lower-class women who are almost certainly the ones to serve as surrogates for upper-middle-class or professional women, the distribution is not fair. This argument does not rebut the charge that it is paternalistic to prohibit women from being paid to be surrogates. Rather, it identifies considerations of justice as a higher value, one that may tolerate a certain amount of paternalism in public policy.

"Another objection to this argument points to considerations besides paternalism. Our capitalistic society already embodies many commercial arrangements in which a lower social class works for relatively low pay, providing services for a higher social class. Examples include domestic service, custodial work, and a range of other occupations. Since we already tolerate many such arrangements, this objection goes, why should it not be acceptable in surrogate motherhood?

"Whether these social arrangements should be construed as a form of class exploitation is a debate that lies well beyond the scope of my presentation to the task force this evening. But the already existing circumstances in which lower classes provide services for better-off members of society does not supply the basis for an argument that it is morally acceptable to create more such arrangements. The form of that philosophical argument is a variation of the attempt to derive an 'ought' from an 'is': 'Because things are this way, it is morally permissible to continue in this way.' If society is to achieve moral progress, that form of argument must be rejected.

"Some feminists have provided a curious twist to the debate about commercial surrogacy. They argue that the standard $10,000 fee paid to a surrogate mother is too *low*, that it is exploitive precisely because it is not a fair wage for services rendered. They calculate that in terms of an hourly wage, based on nine months of twenty-four hours per day of pregnancy, that fee comes to about $1.54 per hour.[36] The proposal to calculate a fair wage for surrogacy on an hourly basis has all the marks of a reductio ad absurdum.

"The potential for better-off women to exploit those who are less well off is the first argument in support of the position against commercial surrogacy arrangements. The second is a broader argument that applies to other biomedical concerns as well. Medical and other health services are a special sort of social good, one that should not be subject to the same market forces that govern the sale of pork bellies. The human body, its parts, and its reproductive products are not 'mere meat.'[37] The United States Congress has wisely enacted a law prohibiting commercial arrangements for procuring and distributing organs for transplantation.[38] There is sufficient evidence of greed, corruption, and duplicity on the part of persons in financial markets, among defense contractors, local and federal officials, and others in the public and private sectors to make us wary of allowing commercial practices to invade and dominate the delivery of health care. Medical services and other health-related activities should not be treated as commodities.[39] To do so is to feed the coffers of profiteers and enrich brokers and middlemen, people eager to reap personal gain from the misfortune of others. Commercial arrangements drain monetary resources away from the direct provision of medical services and products to those in need.

"From all the considerations enumerated here, I conclude that it is not the practice of surrogate motherhood itself that is ethically wrong but, rather, its commercialization. This conclusion answers no to the question of whether there is something intrinsically unethical about surrogacy. It cannot be seen to violate any fundamental moral principle prohibiting certain types of action. But this conclusion does not yet answer the separate question of whether, on the whole, the bad consequences of allowing this practice outweigh the good ones. There is not enough evidence at this point for an empirically well-confirmed answer to that question.

"Of course, we've already heard the objection, if commercial surrogacy is prohibited, isn't it almost certain to result in the disappearance of the practice? Who will come forward to serve as surrogate mothers—except for a few women who want to help their own sisters or daughters or even mothers?

"My reply to this question is simple. The argument that there is nothing inherently unethical about surrogacy is not an argument that surrogacy is a good thing and should therefore be encouraged or promoted. It is simply an argument that noncommercial surrogacy is morally *permissible* and should therefore not be prohibited. If the practice disappears for lack of monetary incentive for women to act as surrogates, so be it. In the absence of evidence or arguments that surrogacy is such a desirable practice that its disappearance would constitute a harm or wrong to society, its loss should not be lamented.

"The argument that surrogacy is a morally flawed activity because of exploitation or the base motives of participants does not stand up to critical analysis. The moral flaws are tied to the commercial features of surrogacy, not to the arrangement itself. Although there is nothing ethically wrong, in principle, with surrogate motherhood, the practice still needs to be evaluated in terms of its good and bad consequences. If it becomes evident that surrogacy arrangements result in more overall harm than benefit, we shall have to conclude that the practice is morally wrong." Teddi closes her presentation on this note.

"You've all given us a lot to think about," Maura remarks. "Any comments or questions?"

"Yes," Jeanne Lodge replies. "I haven't heard enough about the children born of these surrogacy arrangements. Are there any data on that? There must be some information that can help us determine whether surrogacy will really be harmful to the children."

"I've tried to find some such reports, but there don't seem to be any," Tod Nielsen answers. "But Jeanne's question brings us to another point. People are always worried about the bad consequences for these children, but don't forget that these are children who wouldn't have been born at all were it not for the surrogacy arrangement. How can we worry about the possibility of harm to a person who wouldn't otherwise exist?"

"I didn't think we'd be engaging in metaphysics on this task force."

"No, I'm being serious. It's a question of comparing two possible states of affairs. In one state of affairs, child X doesn't exist at all. In the second state of affairs, child X exists and suffers some psychological problems as a result of being born of a surrogate mother. Which state of affairs is better?"

"That's metaphysics, all right. 'Possible worlds' theory."

"A similar situation often comes up in the hospital," Vera Rodriguez points out. "When we debate whether treatments should be withheld or withdrawn from a severely handicapped newborn, we sometimes ask whether the infant would be 'better off dead.' Aren't we comparing a life with pain and suffering against no life at all in that situation?"

"That's an entirely different matter."

"I don't think it's all that different."

Maura interrupts. "Whether this discussion is metaphysics or not, I think we should move on."

"Wouldn't it help to look at the experience of adoption?" Jeanne Lodge asks. "There are books and articles saying that adopted children have a greater than average chance of developing emotional problems."

Tod Nielsen responds: "As I tried to argue in my presentation, the analogies between surrogacy and adoption are unhelpful."

"I agree," Timothy Reardon asserts. "In the case of adoption a child already exists and needs a loving family environment. 'A child is placed for adoption because of the circumstances of the mother which prevent her from caring for the child. Her concern for the child's welfare seeks a permanent and stable home for her offspring.'[40] In this surrogacy business, a woman creates a child for the express purpose of giving it away. The analogy with adoption should be abandoned."

"But we can still try to research the question of whether children who aren't reared by their natural mother suffer more harm than children who are."

"I don't like the term 'natural' mother. It implies that an adoptive mother is 'unnatural,'" Goldwoman complains.

"This meeting appears to be deteriorating into semantic quibbles," O'Brien states. "The hour is late, and I think it's time to adjourn. Before we meet again, please review the different policy options the staff has drawn up in the outline. These can be broadly grouped into five categories: static, private ordering, inducement, regulatory, and punitive. The static approach involves no legislation, leaving the resolution of controversies to a case-by-case consideration in the courts. The private-ordering approach allows the state to validate private arrangements; it would, in essence, facilitate individual surrogacy arrangements. Inducement approaches validate the parties' underlying intentions or agreements only if their actions meet certain statutory requirements. The regulatory approach would create an exclusive mechanism by which an activity such as surrogacy can be carried out. Finally, the punitive approach would impose sanctions on any of a number of different surrogacy practices."[41]

"Do you need a ride?" Teddi Chernacoff asks Roberta Bernstein.

"I'd love one."

As Teddi turns the key in the ignition, Roberta sighs. "You know, I can't help thinking that some of the issues we're discussing here shouldn't have such a high priority from a public policy perspective."

"What do you mean?"

"I'm thinking about AIDS. We're seeing more and more HIV-infected women coming to the hospital pregnant. They're the ones who shouldn't be having babies. The issue of children born of surrogacy arrangements is a trivial one compared with the problem of babies infected with AIDS by their mothers during pregnancy."

Counseling HIV-Infected Women

"Hmmm," Chernacoff muses as she pulls out of the parking lot. "You think it's immoral for HIV-infected women to have babies?"

"Yes, I do," Bernstein asserts.

"I'm surprised to hear you say that," Chernacoff says. "You didn't speak up at the meeting against the morality of women acting as surrogates."

"That's because I don't think it's harmful to the children to be brought into the world in surrogacy arrangements. In all probability, they'll turn out to be normal, healthy infants. But bringing babies into the world who will acquire AIDS is an entirely different matter. Did you ever see any of those babies? It's truly horrible. I've been serving as a consultant on the obstetric and pediatric units caring for AIDS patients. I can tell you, it's one tragedy after another."

"I don't doubt that for a minute."

"You know," says Bernstein, "an HIV-infected woman has up to a 30 percent chance of transmitting the virus to her infant. But even if the baby is lucky and doesn't become infected, it has a 100 percent chance of being orphaned. What kinds of prospects are those?"

"It depends on who's looking at the chances," responds the bioethicist. "Last week a pregnant woman who knew she was going to die of AIDS was being counseled by our AIDS team. When the counselor told her her baby had a 30 percent chance of getting the disease from her, she replied: 'That's the best odds I've heard in a long time.' In situations like this, it really depends on whose perspective we consider."

"Perhaps these women could be helped to adopt a different perspective. After all, if people are doing something immoral, it's appropriate to try to get them to change their behavior or their attitude. That's one of the things counselors are supposed to do."

"That depends on your view of the role of counselors. In genetic counseling, for example, I always thought the counselor was supposed to be nondirective."

"I guess you're right about that. I was thinking of my role as a psychologist. Much of the counseling we do in the mental health field is value-laden. The whole idea behind 'directive' counseling is to get a patient or client to change undesirable behavior patterns."

"Now I see where we appeared to disagree," nods Teddi. "I was assuming a counseling context in which there is no clear right or wrong. In those situations a counselor's function is to provide accurate information and answer questions. It could also include providing emotional support. But in your experience as a psychologist, there are many situations in which it's clear what sort of behavior is good or bad for a client. So, nondirective counseling is appropriate in ethically ambiguous situations, and directive counseling is acceptable when there is a clear right or wrong."

"I accept that analysis," agrees Roberta.

"Now let's come back to HIV-infected women having babies. Is there a clear right or wrong in this situation?"

"As far as I'm concerned, there is."

Teddi ponders for a moment. "Quite frankly, I'm not convinced that it's immoral for HIV-positive women to have children. Let's hear your argument."

"Teddi, you can argue circles around me, you know that, but here goes. The main reason I think it's immoral for HIV-positive women to have babies is the bad consequences for the children who develop HIV infection. There are other considerations as well, but this is the main reason."

"I've heard that sort of argument before. In fact, it's been advanced in the context of genetic disease. The argument has three parts: first, that we should try to provide every child with a normal opportunity for health; second, that in doing so it's not wrong to prevent possible children from existing; and third, that this obligation may require us to refrain from childbearing.[1] I don't want to dismiss the argument without further reflection, but I do think the degree of likelihood that the disease will occur is critical. Some experts cast doubt on the percentage you cited of those who will go on to develop full-blown AIDS. Early statistics tended to support a figure as high as 50 percent, but more recent evidence suggests that the figure may be lower than 30 percent."

"My argument stands regardless of the exact statistic. I'm basing it on a principle you often cite: the 'harm' principle: 'It is justifiable to interfere with people's freedom of action in cases where harm to innocent persons is likely to result.' Is that it?"

"That's close enough. But there are many refinements to that principle, as you know."

"I know, but I'm using it here to justify my view that it's ethically acceptable to try to convince HIV-positive women that they shouldn't have children. Bringing children into the world who are likely to contract a horrible disease, with much suffering and early death, sounds like harm to me."

"But it *is* relevant that fewer than half of the children born of HIV-infected women will get AIDS. As you stated the harm principle, it's wrong to bring children into the world who are *likely* to suffer harm. Again, the *degree* of likelihood is relevant."

"You may be right about that. You're focusing on the likelihood of harm, while I'm emphasizing the magnitude of harm."

"Fair enough. I hate to bring it up again, but remember the discussion at the task force meeting about comparing potential harm to a child with the only alternative—not being born at all? Some committee members wanted to avoid such excursions into metaphysics, but as a philosopher I rather enjoy them. Anyway, the same point holds here as it does in the surrogacy context. How can you weigh the harm to a child of getting AIDS against the child's nonexistence?"

"I think there are fates worse than death, and this is one of them," says Roberta. Getting AIDS as an infant or young child is worse than never having been born at all. We make genetic counseling and prenatal diagnosis available to couples so they can make an informed choice about whether to have a child with birth defects. If it were always preferable to have a life, no matter how much suffering is involved, medicine and public policy wouldn't provide the option of prenatal diagnosis and termination of pregnancy. And you as an ethicist wouldn't support it."

"There are two points in reply to your analogy with genetic counseling and prenatal diagnosis. The first is that those choices are given to women or couples for their own sake, not for the sake of the child who would otherwise be born with handicaps. It's often pointed out by disabilities advocates that one rarely hears a handicapped person say she wishes her parents had decided to abort her. Prenatal diagnosis and the choice to abort a handicapped fetus are practices designed to benefit the parents, not the child. The second point in reply to your analogy is that you've contradicted your own position. In genetic counseling it's precisely the fact that a couple is informed and allowed a free choice of whether to continue the pregnancy or undergo a termination that characterizes the way that sort of counseling is done. Do you think the neutral approach to genetic counseling is misguided and ought to be abandoned? There's an issue of consistency here."

"I told you you could argue circles around me. Now I'm confused. Must I be consistent in either supporting or rejecting nondirective counseling in both cases: pregnant women with AIDS and those carrying a fetus with genetic disease?"

Chernacoff smiles. "Consistency is a virtue, but when there are relevant differences between situations, the same practice may not be appropriate. Let's go back to a distinction we glossed over. Is it your view that HIV-infected women should be counseled to avoid becoming pregnant in the first place? Or that once pregnant, they should be counseled to seek an abortion?"

"To be honest, I hadn't really thought through that distinction. My point is that as clinicians we have an obligation to promote the likelihood of healthy babies. But now I see an important distinction between genetic counseling and counseling HIV-infected women. A pregnant woman is counseled, undergoes an amniocentesis, and learns that the fetus has a genetic anomaly. The woman may choose to abort that fetus and become pregnant again, in the hope of having a healthy baby. The possibility of detecting anomalies in utero allows the woman to abort an unhealthy fetus and carry a healthy one to term. But HIV infection can't be detected in utero, so it's impossible for an HIV-infected woman to make the informed choice to have only healthy babies."

"Do you think a woman who discovers she's carrying an infant with Tay-Sachs disease should choose to abort the fetus?"

"Yes, I think that's the ethically right thing to do. That's a very good analogy with a pregnant woman who's HIV-positive."

"What if the woman with the Tay-Sachs fetus is an Orthodox Jew and opposed to abortion?"

"Well, of course I don't think she should be forced to have an abortion. You know I'm a staunch supporter of reproductive freedom. It's a long way from counseling to coercion. By the same token, I think HIV-infected women shouldn't be coerced into having abortions or avoiding pregnancy in the first place. I'm only talking about counseling people, giving information and advice. Not coercion. Don't back me into a corner. I'm unalterably opposed to mandatory abortion or sterilization."

"I entirely agree with your distinction. All too many people mistakenly conflate coercion with directive counseling or giving advice. In my view, an attempt at rational persuasion doesn't count as coercion."

"Then we do seem to agree on at least two points—that coercing HIV-infected women not to have babies would be wrong, and also that counseling is not a form of coercion. Am I right?"

"I agree with those statements. Where, then, do we disagree?"

"I still maintain that HIV-positive women should be counseled to avoid becoming pregnant. That's in line with the recommendation of the Centers for Disease Control that such women should 'defer' pregnancy. But 'defer' here is a euphemism, since once you're seropositive, you're seropositive for life. I take it that in your view it's wrong to use directive counseling."

"Before I come to a firm conclusion on that, Roberta, I have to ask you another question. Does it work? Everything I've heard suggests that attempts to counsel, persuade, or otherwise influence HIV-positive women not to become pregnant have failed. Even women who have had one or more babies with full-blown AIDS have gone on to get pregnant again. I have in mind the ethical maxim 'Ought implies can.' Before you exhort someone to act in a certain way, it must be possible for the individual to act in that way. If HIV-infected women are incapable of altering their behavior, then it makes no sense to counsel them to do so."

"I don't think we have enough evidence to conclude that counseling never works. There is only anecdotal evidence that some infected women keep getting pregnant, and I think many of those are crack addicts whose behavior is totally out of control. We just don't have adequate studies to demonstrate whether counseling is effective or not."

"Counseling women about pregnancy raises another problematic issue. I've heard some people argue that social context is a relevant factor in determining whether it's immoral for HIV-infected women to have babies. This argument holds that it would be okay to recommend to middle-class or educated HIV-infected women that they not have children, whereas it would not be okay to recommend to poor, minority women that they not have children. Distinctions between social class or race can be justified, according to this viewpoint, even though it's a form of discrimination. It treats one group of women in one way but prohibits treating another social class or racial group of women the same way."

"Yes, I've heard that view expressed," Roberta acknowledges. "It rests on some underlying presumptions for grouping women according to social context. The first presumption is a psychosocial consideration: poor, minority women have so little else in their lives that it is better for them to have children than not to have children. This leads to the conclusion that they should be allowed to decide on their own, without recommendations or directive counseling, whether to have children. The second presumption is more political: poor, minority women are controlled so much by the larger society—by whites, by men, and generally by people with greater wealth and power—that they deserve to be allowed to make all reproductive choices without being influenced in any way. Then there's a third presumption, which I guess is both political and psychosocial: if directive counseling and recommendations were made to middle-class or educated women, they'd still be free to decide for themselves whether to have children, whereas poor, minority women would be 'coerced' by such influences."

"Very interesting," Teddi replies. "But don't you find that argument paternalistic with regard to poor, minority women?"

"I didn't say I accept the argument. But why do you say it's paternalistic? A position that argues *against* directive counseling would seem to permit maximum self-determination for poor, minority women. So in what way is it paternalistic?"

"The paternalistic aspect is those underlying presumptions you mentioned before. They presume to know what's best for a group of women, taken as a group—not as individuals. They also presume to judge how women as a group are likely to react. Middle-class women are capable of exercising free choice; lower-class or minority women aren't. Don't you find that a bit demeaning?"

"The viewpoint is demeaning, but without some factual data to go on I can't assess whether it's true or not."

"There's also a question of justice involved here. I would argue that an unacceptable form of discrimination is embedded in the position that social context calls for different treatment. The discriminatory feature is the principle: 'Treat white, middle-class, HIV-infected women differently from poor, minority, HIV-infected women.' From the standpoint of justice, that's discrimination."

"What's your definition of justice?"

"In situations like this, it's the meaning of justice that says: 'Treat like cases alike; treat different cases differently.' The argument turns on the question of whether social context is a *relevant* similarity or difference with respect to HIV-infected women. I think reasonable people are likely to disagree on this point. The alleged difference between these two groups of women that's taken to be relevant is the value they attach to demonstrating their fertility and having children. Does that value really distinguish poor, minority women as a group from middle-class, white, better-educated women? If that were the case, it might count as a morally relevant reason for making a distinction. We could then justify treating different groups differently, allowing for directive counseling about having children for one group but not for the other."

"I like your analysis, Teddi, but I doubt whether such general values can accurately be attributed to women as members of a social or economic group. It's certainly true that some HIV-infected women come from a cultural background that places a high value on having children. But it's also true that individual women from other social and cultural backgrounds strongly desire children. We have only to look at the many women seeking treatment for infertility, and the whole surrogacy business, to confirm this supposition. Beyond these casual observations, is there any sociological evidence? Have there been claims made by women who are spokespersons for these groups? If so, who are they, and on what basis can they be said to 'represent' the group? There are lots of self-appointed spokespersons for all sorts of groups. We have an example on the task force in Andrea Goldwoman, who acts as though she speaks for all women. Until these questions are answered satisfactorily, I'd have to conclude that there is no fair basis for discrimination between the two groups of women."

"Good, Roberta, we do agree on this. And you've hit on the correct notion of justice here, justice as fairness. We're in agreement in rejecting the position that the social context of HIV-infected women should make a difference in the question of whether it's immoral for them to have children. If it's immoral for one group, it's also immoral for the other."

"Somehow I lost track of our original discussion. Earlier, I thought we disagreed about whether HIV-infected women should be counseled not to have children."

"I said I wasn't entirely certain about that. In fact, I said I wasn't certain whether it's wrong for HIV-infected women to have children. There are two related but distinct questions here: whether it's immoral for these women to have children, and whether directive counseling is ethically right. What we've now agreed on is that whichever way one social or economic group is treated, other social and economic groups should be treated similarly. But we've also agreed on something else: that whatever influence directive counseling and explicit advising have on people, making such recommendations should not be considered a form of coercion. Since coercion is morally wrong, and if directive counseling about childbearing does *not* count as coercion, this leaves open the possibility that it is ethically permissible. However, saying that it's ethically permissible is not to say that directive counseling of HIV-infected women is ethically obligatory."

"But saying only that directive counseling is ethically permissible doesn't give clear guidance to professionals who do the counseling."

"That's true. To say that something is ethically permissible says that it's neither ethically required nor ethically prohibited. But that's not to say nothing at all."

"Huh?"

"I mean," Teddi smiles, "that it leaves it up to the counselor to decide. Physicians, psychologists, nurses, social workers, and others who counsel patients or clients have to use ethical judgment as well as clinical judgment in their professional practice."

"I like that. To emphasize the role of professional judgment and the desirability of maintaining professional autonomy, at a time when that view is rapidly diminishing, is a good thing. So long as you're prepared to accept the ethical permissibility of directive counseling, I'm comfortable with that position. But there's another factor we haven't even discussed."

"What's that?"

"The costs to society in caring for children with AIDS. Couldn't this be a justification for recommending to HIV-infected women that they 'defer' childbearing?"

"Roberta, I'm happy to see we're almost at your house. This 'cost to society' argument is one of my pet peeves in discussions about ethics and public policy. Let me give you the short answer now. It's my contention that the financial cost to society is an insufficiently weighty factor to support a recommendation to a woman that she limit her reproductive choice by not having children. Furthermore, such a recommendation is inconsistent with other practices and policies that support reproductive freedom. To take one example, middle- and upper-middle-class women with high-risk pregnancies are encouraged and supported by the obstetric profession in their quest to have children, despite the actual or potential 'costs to society.' And to go back to the example we've already discussed, the traditional stance in genetic counseling has been nondirective, even after a prenatal diagnosis that reveals a fetus with mental or physical impairments. If a couple chooses to have a child they know will have some handicaps, the cost to society does not count as a moral argument against their decision. My point here is that an argument based on 'costs to society' resulting from the birth of infants with AIDS is inconsistent with other practices and policies. And what's even more troubling, accepting the argument in the context of AIDS can set us on the infamous slippery slope."

"Oh no, not the slope again!"

"You joke. But remember, when it comes to reproductive freedom, we are less secure than we thought we were a few years ago. I would have thought that *Roe v. Wade* settled things once and for all, but you see what's happened recently. Only constant vigilance can protect women against erosion of their reproductive rights and limits on their procreative liberty. This is one of the reasons why I object to drawing the conclusion that it's immoral for women with HIV infection to have children. It's also what bothers me so much about Andrea Goldwoman's rejection of the new reproductive technologies. Her position is rooted in ideology rather than in the world of social and political reality."

"That's exactly the argument she makes against us liberal feminists."

"You're right," Teddi agrees. "Well, one person's real world is another's fantasy. Or something."

"That's my house just ahead, on the left. Thanks for the lift. I guess when we come to our task force recommendations, we'll agree on whether egg donation programs and surrogacy clinics should screen potential donors, recipients, and surrogates for AIDS."

"Absolutely."

"Thanks again. See you soon."

Larry Roberts takes a sip of his morning coffee. "You know," he muses, "it's going to cost us big bucks to hire a surrogate. The going rate is $10,000, and that's only what we pay the woman. Then there are her medical bills and the fee to the broker. Before we're through, we'll have to shell out $25,000 or probably more. We can't afford it."

"Do we have to hire a surrogate?" Bonnie wondered. "The ethicist said paying money to a surrogate isn't ethical. Do you think we could find someone willing to do it for nothing? Or is that illegal?"

"Who knows what's legal or illegal in this surrogacy mess, let alone ethical? Remember, Professor Blackstein told us the laws are changing all the time." Larry thinks for a moment.

"Bonnie, this is a long shot, but I wonder if my sister Frannie might be willing to be a surrogate mother for our baby. Remember how she sympathized with us when we went through the adoption business, then the infertility workups?"

"She certainly was sympathetic, I agree. But it's a big thing to ask of her. What if she feels obligated to say yes but doesn't really want to do it?"

"She's a grown woman; she can stand on her own two feet."

"I don't know, Larry. She could feel obligated to us, and then if she agrees, think how obligated we'd be to her."

"We've been pretty close all our lives. In my family we do things for each other because of our feelings, not because of obligations."

"There's another problem. Frannie's never had children. I think these clinics like to use surrogates who have their own children."

"Why? Frannie's been married. Isn't that good enough?"

"They want women who've experienced what it's like to be pregnant."

"I'm still not sure why."

"Well, it's one thing deciding to have your own baby, one you're going to keep. It's another matter to get pregnant with someone else's child."

"That's for the clinic to decide, not us. If Frannie is willing, the clinic will have to approve the plan anyway. Then they'll probably have to interview Frannie. You know, they have a shrink who does that stuff."

"I still feel uneasy about this, but you know your sister better than I do. I certainly like Frannie, don't get me wrong. But you'll have to do the asking."

"Sure, don't worry. Look, Bon, the worst that can happen is Frannie will say no. Right? We have nothing to lose by asking."

Larry goes to visit his sister and presents the plan. She's surprised at first, then hesitant. Larry backs off.

"Let's just forget I mentioned it. It was a bad idea."

"No, no. I'm not saying I don't want to do it. You know how much I love you and Bonnie. But it's a pretty big step, deciding to carry a baby for nine months. I have to think about it awhile."

"I shouldn't have asked. We don't want to impose on you. Bonnie was very clear about that. She said you might feel obligated to do this, and that wouldn't be right."

"Larry, give me some time to think about it. Okay?"

"Of course. And by the way, we'd pay all your medical expenses, and time lost from work at the end of the pregnancy, and the costs of anything else that might inconvenience you."

"I'm not worried about that part. I just have to make sure I'm prepared to be pregnant for nine months. Money wouldn't change my life as much as being pregnant."

"Okay, Frannie, take as much time as you like to think about it. And if you have any reservations at all, I don't want you to say yes."

Frannie thinks about her brother's request. She talks to a close friend about it. She inquires of several married friends with children what their experiences were like being pregnant. In the end, she decides to help her brother and sister-in-law realize their deepest desire. Once she's absolutely certain, Frannie calls Larry to tell him so. When Larry informs Bonnie, she is elated, and they call the clinic the next day to set up an appointment.

Bonnie and Larry pick Frannie up and drive to the Fecundity Center on the day of their scheduled appointment. They sit down with Mr. Epstein, the administrator, and explain the agreement they've reached.

Mr. Epstein crosses and uncrosses his legs. "This is a bit unusual for us. We normally provide the surrogate for these procedures, and it is the firm policy of the clinic to provide only a surrogate who is married and who has already borne children."

"Why?" Larry asks.

"First of all, we want a surrogate who has experienced childbirth, for psychological as well as medical reasons. Women who have had successful pregnancies with no complications are a better risk. Also, as you no doubt realize, a woman who already has children of her own is less likely to decide she wants to keep the child she's carrying as a surrogate."

"You don't have to worry about that with me," Frannie says. "I'm doing this for my brother and sister-in-law, so I'll be the baby's aunt. I can see the kid any time I like. I can even babysit."

Epstein continues: "As for the married aspect, we like to play it safe. If a woman is married, we require the husband's consent to her serving as a surrogate. That way there are no unanticipated problems. With an unmarried woman, you never know. She may be unstable—uh, pardon me, Ms. Amiga, no offense intended—or during her pregnancy she may meet a man who objects to the arrangement. We just like to play it safe."

Epstein studies the three. "But in this case, since you've made this arrangement privately, and since you're related, I see no reason why we can't accommodate. You'll have to sign our standard contract, and of course, Ms. Amiga will have to undergo all the medical and psychiatric tests we normally require."

"What about the law?" Bonnie asks. "I know there's no law in this state right now, but what if one gets passed some time in the next few months?"

Mr. Epstein smiles. "No one can predict what the legislature may do. All I can say is, for now and the foreseeable future, we're safe. The bill that's before the legislature says nothing at all about the marital status of surrogates. I'm not a lawyer, but our legal counsel has assured us that we have nothing to worry about under our current operating procedures at the clinic."

Larry thinks again about the information they had gotten from Professor Blackstein. "What about the commercial aspect? If we have to pay the clinic for all the services you provide, wouldn't that be against the law if the legislature were to ban commercial surrogacy?"

"As I understand it," Epstein replies, "a ban on commercial surrogacy would mean that the surrogate couldn't be paid and a broker couldn't be paid. But we're not acting as a broker here. You brought your own surrogate, you won't be paying her or us—beyond the medical and psychological screening and the in vitro procedures—so we wouldn't be breaking such a law, even if one already existed."

Bonnie and Larry are satisfied. Frannie has been sitting silently through the legal discussion. When they complete the interview, all three are enthusiastic about the plan.

The Fecundity Center follows standard practice in screening potential surrogates before embarking on the actual procedures. Frannie Amiga has to undergo a psychiatric evaluation[2] and tests to rule out the presence of syphilis, herpes, gonorrhea, hepatitis, and HIV infection. She is in perfect health and has no reason to suspect that she has any disease. A physician at the Fecundity Center takes a complete medical history, but since Frannie's egg is not to be used for the fertilization, there is little concern about her genetic history. Blood samples are drawn, and Mr. Epstein informs Frannie, Larry, and Bonnie that the clinic will be in touch with them in about two weeks when the results come back from the laboratory. They can then proceed with the in vitro fertilization of Bonnie's egg with Larry's sperm.

Two weeks elapse. The secretary at the clinic leaves a message for Frannie at work. When Frannie returns the call, the secretary tells her she'll have to come in to receive the results of the tests in person.

"Is anything wrong?" Frannie asks.

"The clinic's policy is not to give out information over the phone. Could you please tell me when you're available for a consultation with Dr. Upton?"

Frannie makes an appointment to see the clinic psychiatrist. When she is shown into his inner office from the waiting room, Dr. Upton asks her to be seated.

"You know about the lab tests we had to do for medical reasons, before we could proceed here. Those were explained to you in advance, weren't they? Well, I'm very sorry to have to tell you some bad news. Ms. Amiga, your blood tested positive for the HIV antibody."

Frannie stares blankly at the psychiatrist.

Dr. Upton assumes his most professional demeanor. "Two different tests were performed, and they indicate that you are infected with the AIDS virus. I'm very sorry."

"You're sorry! You're sorry? Does this mean I have AIDS? That I'm going to die? Can the test be wrong? It's impossible! I'm not gay. I've never shot drugs. It can't be true!"

In less than two minutes, Frannie's expression has changed from disbelief to fear to anger. Then she begins to cry. Dr. Upton tries to calm her, but Frannie only grows more hysterical. The psychiatrist buzzes the secretary and asks her to call Mr. Epstein. When Epstein enters the psychiatrist's office, Frannie is weeping and keeps exclaiming, through her tears, "I'll kill myself. If I have AIDS, I'll kill myself."

Epstein looks at the distraught woman and the doctor, trying to understand what is going on. Dr. Upton simply says: "We did our routine screening, and the patient is HIV-positive." Epstein goes pale. Nothing like this has ever happened before. It's bad news not only for the weeping woman in front of him but possibly also for the clinic. A flood of worst-case scenarios courses through his mind.

Frannie stops crying, but her voice is shrill and her face is tense as she confronts Epstein. "I don't understand this. I come in here to help my brother and sister-in-law have a baby, you do this screening stuff, and hit me with the news that I have AIDS."

Mr. Epstein and Dr. Upton exchange nervous glances. Still angry but thinking more clearly, Frannie struggles to recall what she heard on a television program about AIDS. "People have rights, you know. This disease is different. A doctor can't just tell somebody they have AIDS. They have to be counseled first. I know my rights. You never counseled me," she accuses Dr. Upton. "Now I have to deal with this. I can't let Larry and Bonnie know. Please don't tell them. I'll commit suicide before I'll let myself get skinny and ugly with AIDS!"

Although the Fecundity Center routinely performs psychiatric evaluations of potential surrogates, it has not adopted the practice of providing pretest counseling before doing blood tests for the HIV antibody. The clinic was advised by its lawyer to add HIV testing to the usual series of tests because of an unfortunate case reported in the legal literature. In that case, involving a surrogacy arrangement made among family members, physicians screened the sperm donor for the HIV antibody but not his sister-in-law, who was the surrogate. Neither the biological father nor his wife had known that the wife's sister had been an intravenous drug user almost five years earlier, and this fact was not elicited by the physicians in taking her medical history. Not until she was five months pregnant was the surrogate tested and found to be seropositive. Because the infant was seropositive at birth (which is true of all infants of seropositive mothers, because they have the mother's antibodies), neither the surrogate nor the intended rearing parents wanted to take custody of the baby.[3]

Since this is the Fecundity Center's first positive test result, the matter of posttest counseling has not arisen before. Mr. Epstein is vaguely aware of a state law requiring such counseling but has never thought it would apply to the Fecundity Center. "After all," he later reasons to Dr. Upton, "we're a fertility clinic, not an alternative test site for AIDS."

Dr. Upton sees that Frannie needs more psychiatric help than he can provide at this point, and—given Epstein's evident distress regarding the administrative problems posed by this development—thinks it best to try to persuade Frannie to seek a voluntary admission to the psychiatric floor of Mercy Hospital. Advising her that this doesn't mean she has a mental illness, he stresses the support she will receive and the possibility that some medication may make her feel better. The doctor promises Frannie that her stay will be temporary: "If you enter on a voluntary basis, you can leave on a voluntary basis."

Although that statement is not entirely true, it convinces Frannie. As her mood alternates between anger and depression, she repeats, "I'll kill myself. But first I'll kill the guy who gave me AIDS." Dr. Upton tells Frannie he will inform Larry of the plans for hospitalization and promises once again to keep the HIV information strictly confidential.

When Larry learns that his sister has agreed to a stay on a hospital psychiatric ward, he is stunned, but all his attempts to pry information out of the psychiatrist are to no avail. Bonnie too is shocked. They have never thought of Frannie as having any mental problems. This development is a mystery to them, and they are saddened by what has occurred.

❀

Discouraged but still resolved to pursue the surrogacy option, Bonnie and Larry decide that their only choice now is to take the costly step of purchasing the services of a surrogate through the clinic. They see no reason to doubt the integrity of the clinic or the competency of its personnel. Any doubts they harbor about the ethics of commercial surrogacy are overwhelmed by their desire for a child. "How can our feelings be wrong?" Bonnie asks. They ask Mr. Epstein to go ahead and find a prospective surrogate who might be a suitable match.

The couple calculates the costs. For the surrogacy part alone, there is a $10,000 payment to the surrogate (a quick call to Professor Blackstein assures Larry that $10,000 is the maximum permitted under the proposed statute that would allow paid surrogacy in their state)[4] and an additional $15,000 to the clinic's lawyer for the brokering service. These amounts do not cover the costs of prenatal care for the surrogate once she becomes pregnant, the obstetrician's fee for delivery of the baby, or the cost of hospitalization during labor and delivery. Nor does it include the costs of in vitro fertilization of Bonnie's egg with Larry's sperm and embryo transfer to the surrogate, which are estimated at more than $5,000 for each attempt.[5] They know that even in expert hands, the successful pregnancy rate following IVF is less than 25 percent.

To afford all this, Bonnie and Larry agree to sell one of their cars and take out a short-term, high-interest loan. These are not their only financial worries. Bonnie plans to quit her job to stay home to take care of the baby for at least six months.

After almost three months a potentially suitable surrogate responds to the Fecundity Center's advertisement. Patty Mae Smith fits the typical profile of women who pass through the screening procedures of surrogate matching agencies: she is twenty-seven years old, Protestant, married with two children; she has a high school diploma and works as a secretary, earning $18,000 a year.[6] She and her husband, Nick, have been having trouble making ends meet. They have discussed whether one or both of them should take a second job and are still considering that option when Patty Mae sees the clinic's advertisement in the newspaper.

"Look, Nick, this clinic in town is advertising for women willing to be surrogate mothers. The women get $10,000 for getting pregnant and giving birth to a baby."

"How do they get pregnant?" Nick asks.

"The advertisement doesn't give the details. It just says 'safe medical procedures are carried out by physicians skilled in techniques of human reproduction.' The couple that hires the surrogate pays all medical expenses related to the pregnancy and childbirth."

"Sounds like easy money. I have no objection, but you're the one who would have to get pregnant. Do you really want to do that again?"

"I felt perfectly fine during my two pregnancies," Patty Mae replies. "Better than when I'm not pregnant, in fact, especially with what I have to go through each month."

Nick and Patty Mae agree that surrogacy is a suitable option to enhance their income. Patty Mae calls to the Fecundity Center for an appointment. Before notifying the contracting couple, the clinic conducts initial screening procedures, including an interview with Dr. Upton.

One of the chief reasons for the psychological screening is to ascertain whether the potential surrogate has a history of any psychiatric disorders. Although Dr. Upton does not have Patty Mae Smith's medical record, he does have her employment records and notes a significant absenteeism.

"I see here that you seem to take sick days every month. In January it was two days, in February three, and last May you took five days off for illness. Is it usually the same thing that keeps you home from work?

"I have a lot of headaches. I also feel awfully tired sometimes. But I don't have a fever or anything catching. I just can't concentrate on work when I feel like that."

"Would you say you're moody or depressed at these times?"

Patty Mae thinks it best to be truthful. "Well, I do cry easily. And a couple of times I mouthed off at my boss when I was feeling like that."

"I notice these regular absences from work occur at about the same time each month. Would you say it's a regular pattern?"

"I guess."

"Have you ever consulted a doctor about these symptoms?"

"No, not really. Only once, when I had to bring a medical excuse for not showing up for the word-processing training program."

"Did that doctor offer a diagnosis?"

"What do you mean?"

"Did he give a name for your condition? For example, did he mention periluteal phase dysphoric disorder?"

"Who could remember anything like that? I don't think so."

"Well, of course I have only what you've told me here this afternoon. Your inability to go to work at about the same time each month, your fatigue, headaches, and crying spells—all this suggests a diagnosis of a disorder known as periluteal phase dysphoric disorder.[7] It's our practice here at the clinic not to accept anyone as a potential surrogate if she has a psychiatric disorder."

"Wait a minute. Are you saying I'm crazy or something?"

"No, I don't mean to suggest anything like that. There are many conditions listed in the official psychiatric *Diagnostic and Statistical Manual* that have nothing to do with psychosis, or what you refer to as 'crazy.' Some of these are mood or behavioral disorders. That may be what you have."

"If you're saying I have PMS, I know all about that. Every woman knows about PMS. You don't need a doctor to tell you you've got it. There are even ads on TV for a medicine to take before your period when you feel like I do. I never heard of PMS being a—what do you call it—psychiatric disorder."

"Well, to tell the truth, there's been a lot of controversy over periluteal phase dysphoric disorder or, as most people call it, PMS—premenstrual syndrome. But despite the controversy, it has been tentatively listed as a disorder in the official psychiatric manual."

"What's the controversy?"

"Well, the dispute has really been within the psychiatric profession. As experts working on a revised edition of the *Diagnostic and Statistical*

Manual were progressing, a great conflict arose over the inclusion of a new diagnostic category then called 'premenstrual phase dysphoric disorder.' Some experts who had studied premenstrual syndrome felt that although a specific psychiatric disorder does exist, it occurs relatively rarely. But most of the controversy that followed didn't have very much to do with the diagnostic category or the condition itself. Instead, it concerned feelings expressed by some feminist groups that this particular diagnostic category would be misleading, since it would inappropriately label women as mentally ill. Beyond that, these feminists worried that the label would be attached not only to the dysphoric disorder but to everything else that happens psychiatrically to women. Other experts worried that the diagnosis was not a scientifically proven category. Eventually, the Board of Trustees of the American Psychiatric Association decided that a special section of the manual, Appendix A, would list this and other tentative diagnoses that deserve attention."[8]

"I still don't see how this applies to me, in this situation. Even if I have PMS, why should it matter now? I won't be having my period while I'm pregnant, will I?"

Swayed by Patty Mae Smith's impeccable logic, Dr. Upton agrees that her PMS should not disqualify her from acting as a surrogate. But then Patty Mae expresses a new worry. She asks the psychiatrist for reassurance that he will not reveal her diagnosis to her employer.

"Frankly, Doc, I'd rather have my boss think I'm lazy or skipping work to go downtown shopping than put an idea in his head that I've got a mental problem."

"There's no need to worry, Ms. Smith," Dr. Upton assures her. "We psychiatrists have the greatest respect for confidentiality. Only in very rare cases do we feel we must disclose a diagnosis to someone other than the patient."

"What do you mean, *patient*? I came in here to apply to be a surrogate mother. I'm not sick, and your 'psychiatric diagnosis' doesn't make me sick."

"You're absolutely right, Ms. Smith. Our training as physicians makes us think of anyone who enters our professional office as a patient, but you're right; you're not a patient at this point. I must remind you, though, that if you're accepted as a surrogate and a pregnancy ensues, you will then become an obstetrical patient. Part of our job will be to inform you thoroughly about the risks of insemination or embryo implantation, the pregnancy itself, and the procedures relating to childbirth. We are committed at this clinic to adhere strictly to the laws of informed consent."

"The only risk I'm worried about now is my boss finding out about my 'disorder.'"

"You have my word that it will be kept confidential."

The Fecundity Center notifies Larry and Bonnie that a suitable surrogate has been found and screened. An appointment is made for the three reproductive collaborators to meet. Everything goes smoothly; Bonnie and Patty Mae even discover that they have a mutual friend. Arrangements are made with the clinic's department of reproductive endocrinology to initiate the medical procedures.

The clinic has developed five separate consent forms for the array of medical and technical procedures, plus an additional contract for the surrogacy arrangement.

For Bonnie, a consent form provides information about the risks and side effects of the fertility drugs she will have to take for ovulation induction, in order to produce mature eggs, and of the procedure used to harvest the eggs. The consent form reads as follows:

CONSENT FOR RETRIEVING EGGS

I hereby authorize physicians at the Fecundity Center to retrieve eggs from my ovaries for the purpose of in vitro fertilization using my husband's sperm. I understand that any eggs obtained will be used as described in this consent form.

I understand that I will be asked to take fertility drugs (clomiphene citrate or human menopausal gonadotropins) which may increase the number of eggs I produce. The major side effects are: bloating, lower abdominal pain; cysts may develop in my ovaries (these will disappear).

I understand that I will be tested, at no charge to me, for syphilis, hepatitis, and AIDS. I have been counseled regarding the significance of these tests. I will be informed of any positive test results and understand that they will not become a part of my permanent medical record.

The procedure for obtaining the eggs involves inserting a thin needle into the ovaries through the abdominal wall. The possible risks of this procedure are bleeding from the insertion site or from the ovaries. If complications deemed to be a result of the egg retrieval develop, physicians at the Fecundity Center will provide care to me. There will be no cost to me of medical care for any immediate complications resulting from the procedure.

Patient	Witness	Date

Physician	Date

For Larry, a consent form specifies that before sperm is retrieved for the in vitro fertilization procedure, he will have to provide in advance a semen sample to be screened for infectious diseases. The form also states that he consents to the use of any leftover sperm for research purposes, but that his sperm will not be used for any inseminations or IVF for women other than his wife.

A third consent form, signed by both members of the couple, describes the IVF procedures following egg retrieval and preceding implantation of the preembryo in the surrogate. This form outlines success rates of the technique in general and at the Fecundity Center in particular.

A separate form allows them to choose cryopreservation of extra preembryos, should more than the requisite number of eggs be harvested and successfully fertilized. The form looks like this:

AGREEMENT FOR THE CRYOPRESERVATION
OF PREEMBRYOS

Cryopreservation is the freezing of preembryos which result from the in vitro fertilization process. Such preembryos are later defrosted and transferred to the woman's uterus.

You are potential users of cryopreservation because you may have excess preembryos after completing an in vitro fertilization cycle. When excess eggs are obtained, you must choose one of several options: (1) donate extra eggs or preembryos; (2) discard the extra eggs or preembryos; (3) cryopreserve the preembryos for future use.

If you decide to participate, the preembryos will be stored in the frozen state until such time as the physician responsible for your care determines the appropriate time to transfer the preembryos to the woman's uterus. Some of the preembryos will then be thawed and examined to see if they have survived. If so, they will be transferred to the woman's uterus.

RISKS AND BENEFITS

The potential benefit of cryopreservation is the possibility of establishing a pregnancy without going through an additional egg retrieval procedure. Cryopreservation has been used successfully for several years in cattle with no adverse results. The experience with humans is limited, but there is no evidence of immediate problems in the children born as a result of using frozen preembryos. The long-term effects are unknown.

Under normal circumstances, less than half of all frozen preembryos survive the thawing stage. As with any technique that requires mechanical support systems, equipment failure can occur. While backup systems are available, unforeseen circumstances could occur that are out of the control of the clinic.

If, after thawing, a preembryo does not appear viable, it will not be transferred to the uterus. It is estimated that about 10 percent of women receiving a frozen preembryo will conceive in that attempt.

DISPOSITION OF PREEMBRYOS

In vitro fertilization, preembryo cryopreservation and transfer are new areas in which legal principles and requirements have not been firmly established. We will consider preembryos which are the result of fertilization of the wife's egg by the husband's sperm to be the property of the couple.

The clinic will maintain all frozen preembryos for 30 months from the time of freezing. During this 30-month period we will abide by your wishes regarding disposition of the preembryos. After this time you may ask us to continue to preserve the preembryos for another thirty months, for an additional fee. In case you lose contact with the Center for any reason, we request that you consent to one of the following options for the frozen preembryos:

1. That the preembryos be donated for use by other infertile couples, if otherwise permitted by applicable law.

Yes _____ No _____

2. That the preembryos be utilized in research projects permitted under applicable law.

Yes _____ No _____

3. That the preembryos be destroyed and discarded.

Yes _____ No _____

In the event that your marital status changes through death or divorce, we will consider this agreement completed and exercise the option that you have chosen above.

Your decision whether or not to participate in the cryopreservation program will not prejudice or harm your future relations with physicians at the clinic, or jeopardize any other options you may wish to exercise at the Fecundity Center.

There is a $600 charge for the freezing and storage of preembryos, which will be billed to you after the egg retrieval is performed.

Larry and Bonnie choose cryopreservation and elect option 1, donation of extra preembryos to other infertile couples.

Patty Mae Smith has to sign a medical consent form for implantation of the preembryo, a modified version of the consent form the clinic normally uses in its egg donation program:

CONSENT TO RECEIVING ANOTHER WOMAN'S EGGS

I hereby agree to implantation in my womb of a preembryo resulting from the fertilization in a dish of donor eggs with sperm from the egg donor's husband. I understand that under this arrangement I will be a gestational surrogate for the couple. I have signed a separate consent form outlining the surrogacy agreement.

I understand that I will have to take some hormones prior to implantation in order to synchronize my cycle, thus preparing my uterine lining for implantation of the preembryo. The risks associated with these hormones are minor, and include ——— .

I understand that there is no guarantee that pregnancy will occur. It is estimated from published data from worldwide experience with this procedure that the pregnancy rate is less than 20 percent. (Actual numbers are too small for accurate statistics.) If pregnancy results, there is no guarantee it will be normal or carried to term. If more than one embryo is implanted, more than one baby may develop, resulting in multiple births.

During pregnancy and delivery, the same types of complications can arise as with a child conceived through sexual intercourse. The Fecundity Center will provide diagnostic and therapeutic services to me during the pregnancy.

I agree to be tested for syphilis, hepatitis, and AIDS. The egg and sperm donors will also be tested for these conditions.

I do this voluntarily, and have been informed of the medical and psychological risks of undergoing this procedure.

The surrogacy agreement used by the Fecundity Center, signed by all three collaborators, follows the pattern of most such contracts, including the schedule of fees to be paid the surrogate, clinic, lawyers, physicians, and any other parties involved. Section 4 contains the following provisions:

4. The schedule of fees and payments outlined in this agreement represents compensation for services and expenses, and in no way is to be construed as a fee for termination of parental rights or a payment in exchange for a consent to surrender the child for adoption. In addition to other provisions contained herein, payments shall be as follows:

(A) $10,000 shall be paid to Patty Mae Smith, Surrogate, upon surrender of custody to Lawrence and Bonnie Roberts, the natural and biological parents of the child born pursuant to the provisions of this agreement, for surrogate services and expenses in carrying out her obligations under this agreement.

(B) The fee to be paid to Patty Mae Smith, Surrogate, shall be deposited with the Fecundity Center, the representative of Lawrence and Bonnie Roberts, at the time of signing of this agreement, and held in escrow until completion of the duties and obligations of Patty Mae Smith, Surrogate, as herein described.

(C) Lawrence and Bonnie Roberts, natural parents, shall pay the expenses incurred by Patty Mae Smith, Surrogate, pursuant to her pregnancy, more specifically defined as follows:

(1) All medical, hospitalization, and pharmaceutical, laboratory, and therapy expenses incurred as a result of Patty Mae Smith's pregnancy, not covered or allowed by her present health and major medical insurance, including all extraordinary medical expenses and all reasonable expenses for treatment of any emotional or mental conditions or problems related to said pregnancy, but in no case shall any such expenses be paid or reimbursed after a period of six months have elapsed since the date of the termination of the pregnancy, and this agreement specifically excludes any expenses for lost wages or other non-itemized incidentals related to said pregnancy.

(2) Patty Mae Smith's reasonable travel expenses incurred at the request of Lawrence and Bonnie Roberts, pursuant to this agreement.[9]

In addition to the surrogate's promise to relinquish custody and parental rights at birth, the agreement contains provisions regarding modification of fees in case of miscarriage or stillbirth, or in case the surrogate is found to have behaved in a way that causes a health problem in the child. Also included are a number of specific limitations on the surrogate's behavior during pregnancy, and additional limitations on the surrogate's control over medical decision-making during pregnancy.

The surrogate consent form used by the Fecundity Center goes beyond the usual contracts in that it describes the psychological risks of carrying a pregnancy with the intent to relinquish the baby and the risks of emotional distress following birth and surrender of the child. After the Baby M case and other cases that had achieved notoriety, the clinic wants to take no chances.

Following the IVF and implantation procedures, Larry and Bonnie try to keep their minds on other things for the next two weeks while they await the results of Patty Mae Smith's pregnancy test.[10] They keep reminding themselves that the chances of achieving a pregnancy are less than one in four. Their worst fears are confirmed when the clinic calls to notify them that this attempt has failed. They embark on the same process again, once more with lack of success. At this point, the couple has spent $10,000 for the medical procedures alone, not counting the broker's fee to the clinic and payment to the surrogate in the event a pregnancy is achieved.

They had not counted on these extra expenses, nor did they anticipate the emotional toll the failed attempts would take. Larry and Bonnie begin to blame each other, each alleging the other's biological contribution to the ongoing failure. And, of course, it is easy to lay blame on Patty Mae, in whom a pregnancy has not occurred. Larry telephones the reproductive endocrinologist at the clinic to inquire whether there is anything physically wrong with Patty Mae. The physician informs Larry that her physical examination during the screening procedures revealed nothing abnormal. Had there been any potential problem detected during the screening, she never would have been accepted into the program.

"In any case," the physician cautions, "Ms. Smith is now our patient at the clinic, and we can't really discuss her medical condition with you. That would be a breach of confidentiality."

"Hold on a minute," Larry fumes. "She's only your patient because of us. We have a contract with her and with your clinic. What about our rights?"

"Mr. Roberts, I'm a doctor, not a lawyer. If you wish to know about your rights, I suggest you call the clinic's attorney. The only rights in question at the moment are a patient's right to confidentiality in the physician-patient relationship. And I'm bound to honor that right."

"I'll get my own lawyer if I need to, thanks." Larry thinks he had better not alienate this physician, since he's also the doctor who is taking care of Bonnie. The way things are going, more eggs will have to be harvested from her and fertilized in the dish, and further attempts made at implantation. Larry decides to call the clinic psychiatrist, and Dr. Upton suggests they come in for a consultation. Larry asks if they will have to pay extra for the visit, and the psychiatrist says no; it is part of the service the clinic provides. Larry and Bonnie make an appointment.

In the psychiatrist's office Bonnie's face is puffy from crying, and she is not wearing makeup. Larry keeps his arms folded across his chest and stares straight ahead, never looking at his wife. After a few failed attempts to get them to talk, Dr. Upton suggests that they visit a marriage counselor.

"There's nothing wrong with our marriage," Larry snaps. "It's Bonnie's eggs that are the problem."

"My eggs! How do you know it's not your sperm?" Bonnie bursts into tears.

Bonnie lies awake at night, fitful, anxious, and depressed. In the morning she can barely drag herself out of bed to go to work. When the couple realizes that without Bonnie's salary they will be in even worse financial straits, they decide to seek psychiatric help. The cost of Bonnie's therapy is another unexpected expense but one they feel is necessary.

Two months later, when the clinic calls to say that the latest attempt following in vitro fertilization and embryo transfer is a success, Larry and Bonnie go out to celebrate. They spend the whole dinner discussing babies' names.

Patty Mae's pregnancy proceeds uneventfully, and in the sixteenth week, in accordance with the provisions of the surrogacy contract, an amniocentesis is performed. The relevant provision of the contract reads as follows:

Patty Mae Smith, Surrogate, agrees that she will not abort the child once conceived except if, in the professional medical opinion of the inseminating physician, such action is necessary for the physical health of Patty Mae Smith or the child has been determined by said physician to be physiologically abnormal. Patty Mae Smith further agrees, upon the request of said physician, to undergo amniocentesis or similar tests to detect genetic or congenital defects. In the event said test reveals that the fetus is genetically or congenitally abnormal, Patty Mae Smith, Surrogate, agrees to abort the fetus upon demand of Larry and Bonnie Roberts, natural parents, in which event, the fee paid to the surrogate will be in accordance with paragraph 9 [$1,000]. If Patty Mae Smith refuses to abort the fetus upon demand of Larry and Bonnie Roberts, their obligations as stated in this agreement shall cease forthwith, except as to obligations of paternity or maternity as imposed by statute.[11]

All three parents anxiously await the results of the amniocentesis. After two and a half weeks the clinic calls to inform them that they must appear in person to obtain the results. As the secretary ushers them into the office, she introduces them to a woman none of them has met before.

"This is Ms. McNeil. She's a genetic counselor here at the clinic." Ms. McNeil smiles and invites Larry, Bonnie, and Patty Mae to sit down and make themselves comfortable.

Dealing with Medical Labels

Bonnie glances nervously at Larry. Ms. McNeil scrutinizes the three parents, clears her throat, and begins.

"Thank you all for coming down. We like to discuss things face-to-face with our patients, so we can answer any questions. Now we did the amniocentesis and found no major genetic problems." Ms. McNeil looks back and forth from one to the other. "In fact, your fetus doesn't have any genetic diseases. But I must tell you, we found a minor genetic anomaly."

Bonnie's face tenses up. "I knew it. There's something wrong."

"As I said, it's not a genetic disease. It's called a 'chromosomal aberration.' There is an extra Y chromosome, making a total of 47 rather than the usual 46."

"So what does that mean?" Larry blusters.

"The fetus is male. All the other pairs of chromosomes are normal. But in males, the pair of sex chromosomes normally consists of one X and one Y chromosome. Your fetus has an extra Y chromosome. Frankly, genetic experts disagree about the meaning of this. Some say there is a real risk of mild mental retardation, emotional difficulty, and possibly antisocial behavior in later life.[1] Others say that abnormalities of the sex chromosomes have only a slight effect on mental or physical ability.[2] In any case, children with this chromosomal anomaly appear normal until the age of about twelve—"[3]

"Wait a minute," Larry interrupts. "I remember hearing about this on the news a while back. Isn't this the 'criminal chromosome'"?

"I was about to tell you some of the history surrounding XYY," Ms. McNeil resumes. "Early studies suggested that XYY men were generally much taller than average, and tended to be more aggressive and sexually active than men with the normal XY complement. Researchers also found sex chromosome abnormalities to be relatively common in prisons and in hospitals treating criminals."[4]

"I was right! The criminal chromosome! Our contract provides for an abortion in case the fetus is abnormal. This baby is abnormal, so that's that."

Bonnie appears hesitant, wanting to probe further. She asks the genetic counselor: "Is my husband right? Do you recommend an abortion?"

Ms. McNeil hedges once again. "Well, it's a genetic abnormality, there's no doubt about that. But there isn't any physiologic abnormality, and the evidence for behavioral abnormality is still uncertain. As for an abortion, we genetic counselors don't really make recommendations to couples. We just like to give the facts."

"Well, you've given me all I need to know!" Larry exclaims.

"I'd like to hear more," Bonnie insists. "Tell me about the studies you mentioned."

"I will, but I have to emphasize that this is an area of ongoing controversy and much uncertainty. One reason so much is known about the sex chromosomes of men in prison is that researchers used to have an easy time gaining access to such institutions. This has changed in recent years, but before about 1975 it was common to conduct biomedical and behavioral research in prisons and mental institutions. From 1959—the time of the first report of sex chromosomal anomalies—until 1970, many studies of institutionalized populations were done. A few researchers drew conclusions that XYY men appeared to be 'a unique group of uncontrollable psychopaths.' Later review of those early studies led to serious doubts about the validity of their conclusions. For the most part, the studies were criticized on methodological grounds.[5]

"More recent studies find no physical or behavioral characteristics that distinguish XYY males from others, except perhaps that XYY males are a little taller than XY males.[6] The fact remains however, that more XYY men were found in mental and penal institutions than are present in the population at large, but that can be explained by other theories.[7] Still, though the evidence is weak, there is some correlation between XYY and dullness, or educational retardation. This tends to be explained by a 'developmental lag' in XYY individuals."[8]

"Isn't 'developmental lag' a euphemism for 'retarded'?" Larry asks skeptically.

"It means simply that there is 'a degree of delay in mental and physical maturation.'[9] I think it's fair to say that the whole history of XYY shows it to be a 'socially charged scientific issue.'[10] Although it's quite clear by now that there was very little basis for the claims about a criminal chromosome, 'the conclusion that XYYs were supermales, or doomed to be criminals or superaggressive . . . was publicized as though it were already a scientific conclusion.'[11] Compared to other types of genetic abnormalities, the XYY chromosomal anomaly is quite minor."

"Minor for you, maybe, but not for us. Even if my son won't turn out to be a superaggressive criminal, I don't like the idea of bad genes. You said he would have a 'developmental lag,' and that's bad enough for me," Larry asserts.

"I said he *may* have a delay in physical or mental maturation," Ms. McNeil emphasizes. "It's not inevitable."

"But isn't the point of having an amniocentesis to avoid any abnormalities?" Bonnie asks. "We don't want to take any chances. That's why we had the prenatal diagnosis."

"That's right," Larry asserts. "Wasn't that why we all signed the contract? If the fetus has any defects, the surrogate has to have an abortion."

"Just a second here!" Patty Mae enters the conversation. "I really don't think this extra chromosome is any reason to have an abortion. The contract we signed talked about genetic *diseases*. Ms. McNeil just told us this is only a minor abnormality. Abortion is a serious thing; you can't just go and get an abortion for any old reason."

"Look, Patty Mae," Larry interrupts angrily, "this isn't your decision. You signed a contract. The contract says if the fetus is genetically abnormal, you agree to abort the fetus on our demand. We demand it. Period."

"Well, I'm not going to do anything against my conscience," Patty Mae insists. "It's wrong to abort a fetus for no good reason. I'm in favor of an abortion only if there's a serious defect, or definite mental retardation."

"Well, you have no choice. I don't want to raise a kid who's going to have a chance of being a retard, or maybe end up a criminal."

"Larry, please," Bonnie begs. "Can't you be a little more civil? I think we should look at what the contract actually says. I forget the exact words. Ms. McNeil, do you have a copy of the contract?"

"No, I'm sorry, not here. But I can get one from the office. Excuse me a moment."

As soon as Lois McNeil leaves the room, Patty Mae speaks up. "I know my legal rights. I asked a lawyer about this. My lawyer told me, and I quote, I cannot assign to another person the right to compel me to have an abortion. She said there's a limit to what can be in a contract. Under *Roe v. Wade*, my lawyer said, the state has no constitutional authority to enforce a contract that prohibits me from terminating this pregnancy or that requires me to do so." [12]

Larry stares at Patty Mae. Unable to rebut her legal assertions, he sits in silence. Ms. McNeil enters the room with a copy of the surrogacy contract, and Larry snatches it from her.

"Okay, listen to this. It says here: 'Patty Mae Smith agrees to undergo amniocentesis or similar tests to detect genetic and congenital defects. In the event said test reveals that the fetus is genetically or congenitally abnormal, Patty Mae Smith, surrogate, agrees to abort the fetus upon demand of Larry and Bonnie Roberts, natural father and mother, in which event, the fee paid to the surrogate will be in accordance to paragraph 10.' [13] That sounds clear to me. Ms. McNeil, is this fetus genetically abnormal or not?"

"I would have to say there is a genetic abnormality. An extra Y chromosome is a chromosomal abnormality, and that's genetic."

"Okay, I guess it's settled then," Larry states smugly. "We'll call the lawyer and—"

Bonnie interrupts. "Wait, Larry, there's another option." She is studying the surrogacy agreement. "It says here that 'if Patty Mae Smith refuses to abort the fetus upon demand of Larry and Bonnie Roberts, the obligations of the natural father and mother as stated in this agreement shall cease forthwith, except as to obligations of paternity imposed by statute.' [14] I guess that means we'd have to pay child support or something."

Patty Mae looks surprised. "Pay child support? For what? Not to me! I didn't say I wanted to raise this child. I just don't want to abort it."

At this point, the genetic counselor sees she has little further role to play. She excuses herself and calls in Mr. Epstein, the administrator. Larry confronts Epstein.

"I thought when this clinic provides a surrogate, a psychiatrist performs an evaluation. Did the shrink examine this bimbo? Or what?"

Bonnie becomes nervous at Larry's outburst. She's afraid Mr. Epstein might question Larry's fitness to be a parent and call off the whole arrangement. Recalling their earlier difficulty when the adoption agency uncovered Larry's past psychiatric problem, she is now worried that her husband's volatile nature will lead someone to delve into his past once again. The couple has discovered that old diagnostic labels tend to stick.

Epstein manages to calm Larry down. "Yes, of course Dr. Upton interviewed Ms. Smith. That's part of our screening process here at the clinic. Dr. Upton found her suitable to serve as a surrogate."

"Excuse me, but can I ask what the psychiatrist was supposed to be evaluating in the interview?" Bonnie asks politely.

Patty Mae retorts, "That's none of your business! Psychiatric evaluations are supposed to be confidential." When she sees Bonnie's pained expression, Patty Mae softens. "Sorry, hon, I didn't mean to jump at you. The psychiatrist asked me lots of questions about my children, my marriage, and my feelings. He spent a lot of time on how I would feel about giving up the baby. But you know, I don't remember him asking any questions about how I feel about abortion."

Epstein adds: "Yes, the purpose of the psychiatric interview is to see whether a woman who chooses to become a surrogate understands completely what she is agreeing to. The psychiatrist also looks for signs of any mental or emotional disorder, or some reason why she might not be fit to be a surrogate."

"Well, this is a reason right here," Larry says. "She's not abiding by our contract."

Seeing no progress in the discussion, Epstein suggests that the three parents consult a lawyer, a psychiatrist, or both. Bonnie looks for an amicable way to end the meeting.

"Why don't we go home and think things over for a few days. Larry and I will discuss this, and Patty Mae, you can talk it over with your husband. Then we can meet again in, say, five days and see where we are. If we can't come to an agreement next time, we'll have to consult our lawyers."

"That sounds good to me," Larry says.

"Fair enough," Patty Mae agrees.

Patty Mae flops down on the couch in her living room. "Bad news," she says to her husband. "There's some genetic problem with this baby I'm carrying for the Robertses, and they want me to have an abortion."

"So? What's the problem?" asks Nick. "Wasn't that in the contract you guys signed?"

"How come it's so easy for everyone but me to be so legalistic about the contract?"

"Patty, it's a legal document. There are laws against breaking a contract."

"Yes, but I happen to know they can't force me to get an abortion if I don't want one. When we had the lawyer look over the contract, she told me."

"Well, why don't you want to have an abortion?"

"I wouldn't mind if it was a serious problem."

"What *is* the problem, anyway?"

"An extra Y chromosome."

"How many are there supposed to be?"

"Normal boys have one. This baby has two."

"So what does that do to the baby?"

"It may make it mentally retarded, and there's something else about maybe becoming a criminal. The counselor was very iffy about it all. She didn't seem sure herself. But the Robertses—especially Larry—were certain they didn't want a baby who might grow up abnormal in some way."

"I don't blame them, Pat. But wait a sec. What happens to our money?"

"*Our* money?"

"Oh all right, *your* money. But remember, we both agreed to go through with this. What happens to the ten thousand bucks? Does it go down the drain? Where's that contract? I want to see what it says about the money if there's an abortion."

"I know what it says, Nick. I'll get $1,000."

"That sure is a lot less than $10,000."

"I know, but I don't feel right about aborting a fetus with a minor problem. And it has nothing to do with the money."

"What happens if you refuse, and decide to go through with the pregnancy?"

"They won't have to pay the $1,000 either. But they would have to pay child support."

"To us? Patty, I never agreed to have another child! The plan was for you to be a surrogate mother and give the baby to the Robertses. That's all I agreed to."

"I suppose we could give the baby up for adoption."

"Then we get no money at all. No $10,000, no $1,000, no nothing. No way! I think you should have the abortion and get it over with. Then maybe you could try again as a surrogate. That way, we'd get a grand this time and, if everything goes okay, ten grand next time. Even more than we bargained for."

"Hmmm. I don't know."

"Look, Pat, here's another thing. If you start all over again and get pregnant, you won't have to deal with PMS for another nine months. Remember how bad that was? You're forgetting now, because you've been pregnant for the past four and a half months."

"That's the best reason I've heard so far. I'm not really that opposed to abortion. I think you're right, though. It's best for everybody if I go ahead and get an abortion."

Patty Mae calls the Robertses to tell them her decision, and they are relieved. When Patty Mae broaches the subject of another try, Larry says, "Sure, sure. Give us a call when everything's taken care of. Meanwhile, I'll let the clinic know." Larry telephones Mr. Epstein, who informs him that he and Bonnie will have to consult with Dr. Furillo, the reproductive endocrinologist at the clinic who does the medical procedures. Larry leaves a message for the specialist to call him back.

The physician telephones Larry later that day. "Mr. Roberts? This is Dr. Furillo calling. I'm sorry things didn't work out for you this time. How can I help you?"

"Thanks for calling back, Doc. My wife and I would like to try again, but we don't know if that's possible with the same surrogate. I guess they told you the fetus has an extra Y chromosome. We just couldn't handle it, and Patty Mae's going ahead with the abortion, like the contract says. Is there some way she could have caused this? I mean, we want to try again, but not if there's a chance that something will go wrong again the next time."

"Of course, Mr. Roberts, there's always a chance that something can go wrong. But this particular chromosomal anomaly happens by chance; it's an error in cell division. The chances of its happening a second time are very small."

"How small is small?"

"The frequency per thousand in live-born births in the general population for XYY is 1.5."[15]

"I think I understand what that means. But what about a different problem, though? If something went wrong one time with this surrogate, isn't there a greater chance of another kind of problem with the chromosomes?"

"To be honest, Mr. Roberts, very little is known about the causes of these things. I can assure you, though, that the problem isn't with the particular surrogate you've chosen."

"Does that mean the problem is with me or my wife? Is that what you're saying, Doc? I want you to be straight with me."

"I'm telling you all I know about these kinds of chromosomal accidents, Mr. Roberts. But you shouldn't think of blaming anyone."

"Does that mean we could use Patty Mae again as a surrogate?"

"That would be up to her, of course, Mr. Roberts. I'll have to discuss the matter with Ms. Smith, who is my patient, too, as you know. But I can tell you that a delay of several months may be necessary before Ms. Smith will be ready, from a medical point of view, for another attempt at embryo implantation."

"Okay, Doc, thanks a lot for calling. I'll tell my wife everything you said. Thanks again."

❧

When Larry informs Bonnie about the conversation with Dr. Furillo, she is disconsolate.

"Oh, Larry, I couldn't stand to go through another waiting period. I'm sure I'll get depressed again."

"Do we have any choice?"

"We could try to get another surrogate. The clinic is always placing ads for surrogates. I'm sure they can find another one for us."

"We'll still have to wait. Either way, it's not going to happen immediately."

"I can't take much more of this, Larry. I can't take much more."

"I know it's hard, Bon, but we have to hang in there."

"Larry, there's another thing. I don't feel right about using the same surrogate after there's been a problem."

"The doctor told me the problem wasn't with her. That makes sense. After all, it was your egg and my sperm. I hope the problem isn't with us."

"I just think it would be bad luck, that's all. I'd like to get a fresh start."

"Maybe you're right.

"I'd feel better about starting all over with a new surrogate."

"I'm not sure it makes sense, but whatever you say. You want me to call the clinic?"

"Yes, please."

Larry telephones Mr. Epstein and informs him of their decision to try again with another surrogate. Epstein is agreeable and begins the search for a new surrogate. He then has the unpleasant task of telling Patty Mae Smith that the Robertses wish to find a different woman for their next attempt at surrogacy. Preoccupied with thoughts of the forthcoming abortion, Patty Mae takes the news calmly.

Three months after her abortion Patty Mae experiences a return of her PMS symptoms, which appear to be worse than before. One evening her husband comes home from work to find her sprawled on the couch, watching TV and eating potato chips.

"No dinner?"

"Nick, I just got home half an hour ago. I'm beat!"

"Why don't we go out to Burger King or order a pizza?"

"Nick, I'm hungry after working all day. Besides, I don't want to give the kids junk food for dinner."

"Well, what do you expect me to do? Hire a full-time cook?"

Patty Mae begins to sob. "I don't know, this PMS is getting me down."

"You can say that again! You're tired. You're hungry. You're depressed. You're pissed at me. It's always something."

"I'm not doing it on purpose, you know. I can't help it."

"Did you ever think of going to a doctor?"

"I asked some of the girls at work. Jenny said she knew a psychiatrist who treats PMS."

"Patty, I know you're moody and irritable, but you're not crazy! Why do you think you need a shrink?"

"I didn't say I was crazy! I said there was a psychiatrist who treats PMS. It doesn't mean you're crazy if you go to a psychiatrist for treatment."

"What do you have to do? Lie on a couch?"

"Are you being sarcastic?"

"I'm just asking."

"I guess the psychiatrist will give me some pills."

"You already have pills. Didn't you get the ones we see on the TV ads all the time?"

"Yes, but you can get those in any supermarket. A psychiatrist would write a prescription for something stronger."

"Yeah, so then you'll be a druggie. Is that what you want?"

"All I want is to get some relief, that's all."

"Isn't there some other kind of doctor who can help? One who deals with female problems?"

"Maybe, I'll have to find out. I'll call Jenny and see what she knows."

❀

Patty Mae learns that a local feminist organization sponsors a support group for women with PMS. She calls, and is given the name of one woman who has received medical treatment for PMS and another who has undergone psychiatric treatment. Each woman swears by the treatment she received. Confused, Patty Mae decides to attend a session of the support group, which meets on Monday nights at the Unitarian Church. Like most of the women there, the group leader, Mary Liston, has experienced PMS herself. She opens the meeting by introducing three invited participants.

"Welcome, everyone. I see a number of new faces this evening, along with many of our regulars. Tonight we're going to depart from our usual format of sharing our personal experiences. Those of you who were here about a month ago will remember that we decided to invite a couple of people with special expertise to bring their perspectives on PMS, and to help settle some disagreements that arose among members of our group. So we'll begin the meeting with a few brief presentations by our invited guests. Then we'll be open for questions and discussion. We're lucky to have Althea Jefferson, an attorney who has represented women with severe PMS in criminal trials, and Laura Gordon, a sociologist who has done research on how the medical model is applied to ordinary life processes such as aging and menopause. Also with us tonight and representing Women against Reproductive Oppression is Andrea Goldwoman, whom many of you know. Andrea will serve as a commentator on the two presentations. If we're ready to start, I'll ask Professor Gordon to begin. Laura?"

"Thank you, Mary, and good evening everyone. I thought I'd share with you some of the findings of research on the medicalization of behavior and show how it applies to PMS. The term 'medicalization' refers to 'the process and product of defining and treating human experiences as medical problems.'[16] In some cases, medicalization is confined to labeling a type of behavior as a disease or disorder rather than considering the behavior as socially deviant, as a variation in the wide array of human conduct. In other instances, medicalization goes beyond labeling and the search for biological causes to a search for medical means of 'treating' the behavior. Let me illustrate briefly with a couple of examples.

"The first example is hyperactivity in children, a condition that has come to be known as 'minimal brain dysfunction,' or MBD.[17] Extensive research over the past twenty years or so has revealed very little about the nature of hyperactivity, and even less about any biochemical or neurobiological causes it may have. There is some vagueness about how to mark the boundary separating MBD children, who are termed 'hyperactive,' from the ordinary variety of very active children. Most children given a diagnosis of MBD have been boys between the ages of six and nine. One difference found through research is that the so-called MBD children respond remarkably well to certain psychoactive drugs. Somewhat paradoxically, these drugs—amphetamines and Ritalin—are stimulants, which have the opposite of a calming effect on most adults. In hyperactive children, however, these drugs not only lower the level of physical activity but also increase the attention span. Finding a drug that can alter behavior in this group of children led researchers who favor the medical model to label hyperactivity a 'disorder' and to consider the administration of drugs a 'therapy.'

"Now I don't want to be misunderstood here. I admit that giving these drugs to children may well benefit them. For example, if children are unable to sit still and concentrate in school, there is no doubt that finding a way to enable them to learn provides a benefit. But a question remains about whether to conceptualize their behavior as a 'disease' or 'disorder' and to construe drugs as 'therapy.' This is my point about the medicalization of behavior.

"A further social critique of the way hyperactivity in children has been handled goes to the setting. 'Diagnosis' and 'treatment' are medical terms. But as applied to hyperactive children, they have been closely linked to the schools. In some cases, hyperactive children who neglect to pop their morning pill have been sent home from school to take their medicine. I agree with the critics who have argued that public schools are not the proper place for the administration of drugs to children. Not only is this one more step in the increasing medicalization of all sorts of socially deviant behavior; it also sends a message that is wrong for our time. Children get the message that popping pills is an acceptable way of affecting mood or behavior, while in another classroom they are bombarded with antidrug propaganda under the guise of drug education. If we are dealing here with a social problem of children who are disruptive in school, or a psychological problem of children who are unable to concentrate, is it really appropriate to look for one more technological fix? That sends the wrong message to the children, misleads society about the power of technology, and also helps to foster the belief that there is an easy solution to complex problems.

"Before turning to PMS, I want to say a few things quickly about an attempt to identify a group of males believed to be at high risk for aggressive behavior and even criminal tendencies because they possess an extra chromosome. This is part of a much larger topic, the search for biological bases of behavior, but I want to draw some analogies with PMS."[18]

At the mention of extra chromosomes, Patty Mae Smith perks up. Her mind has been wandering during a talk that seems to have little relevance to her, but now she listens more attentively to Professor Gordon's words.

"Without going into detail about the genetics, I'll just summarize by saying that some psychiatrists and other scientists believed that having an extra Y chromosome predisposes males to aggressive or violent behavior. Others were unsure but wanted to research the question. One research program involved efforts to identify male infants with the XYY chromosomal abnormality at birth, to observe them in early childhood, and to develop an early intervention program as a 'preventive' measure. An objection raised against this program was the possibility that identifying infants as XYY at birth might serve as a 'self-fulfilling prophecy' regarding aggressive or antisocial conduct on the part of these individuals in later life.[19] When it was suggested that maybe the parents shouldn't be told the exact purpose of the research, critics replied by saying that would be unethical because then the parents wouldn't be giving truly informed consent.

"In the case of both XYY and PMS, medical scientists have looked for the biological roots of socially deviant behavior. Interestingly, in both cases it has been suggested that finding a biological cause of antisocial or aggressive behavior can mitigate the individual's moral responsibility for that behavior. Beyond that, as I think we'll be hearing from Althea Jefferson, biological causes have even been used as a legal defense—based on 'diminished capacity'—for violent criminal acts.

"From my perspective as a sociologist, I think we have to look at the social consequences of putting labels such as XYY or PMS or MBD on people. Will individuals who are so labeled be ostracized? Could such labeling lead to mandatory screening programs, or be used by employers to rule out the hiring of certain people? Most worrisome, I think, is the growing tendency to search for the biological determinants of human behavior. This emphasis detracts attention from the important social problems we need to face and tackle as a society: poverty and the feminization of poverty, unemployment among urban youths, poor inner-city schooling, and the rest. It is well established that almost all human behavior is a product of numerous and complex interacting causes. Genetic determinism is a pernicious idea that will lead to discrimination, ostracism, and possibly even forced intervention into the lives of those found to be 'genetically programmed' to act in certain ways. We have to resist the notion that only by identifying the biological root causes of antisocial or other deviant forms of behavior can we fashion appropriate responses: punishment, therapy, or rehabilitation for criminal offenders, and medical intervention for individuals found to have chemical imbalances or deficiencies believed to cause their aberrant behavior.

"I've spent some time on the details of MBD and XYY to show that the medicalization of behavior is not confined to women but has been used to characterize conditions and behavior in children and in men as well. Now let me turn to a topic closer to the interests of this group—the medicalization of PMS. As I can show rather quickly, PMS has become medicalized.[20] 'Behaviors that previously were identified as the symptoms of neurosis or criminality or the products of women's imaginations are coming to be seen as manifestations of a biological imbalance that can be diagnosed and treated by medical professionals.'[21] In the 1930s it was proposed that the symptoms we now refer to as PMS could be traced to the continued circulation of an excessive amount of female sex hormone in the blood. Later, however, that theory was discredited, and today there is no agreement among medical scientists on the biological causes.

"By the 1940s the use of progesterone replacement therapy as a treatment began in England and became quite popular in the 1950s. By 1981 physicians in the United States were beginning to prescribe it. Without going into the medical literature or the scientific research, I can report that there has been much controversy over this mode of treatment. The major research on progesterone treatment for PMS has been criticized as methodologically unsound, and some critics have argued that both lack of efficacy and questions about long-term safety suggest the need for caution.

"At this point, PMS is becoming institutionalized. There has been a growth of clinics in the United States and England. In both France and England, PMS has been used with success as a legal defense, and similar attempts have been made in American courts. The Boston Women's Health Book Collective has issued a warning, which I endorse wholeheartedly, that it is dangerous to label premenstrual behaviors as hormonally based. They claim that this is a maneuver designed to keep women in their place. It is surely a mistake to promote the view that women are controlled by their hormones. Not only does this view suggest that 'women are biologically unable to perform competently in responsible occupations.'[22] It is also sometimes expressed in the more pernicious belief that when it comes to the propensity for violent behavior, a premenstrual woman can be a 'walking time bomb.'

"Yet I have to admit that some women actually favor the medical model approach to PMS, since it 'serves to legitimate women's experiences by attributing them to hormones instead of hysteria.' We cannot deny that the medicalization of PMS 'is, to some extent, an attempt to improve women's experiences by using modern medical theories, methods, and tools.'[23] Nevertheless, it is up to us as women to decide for ourselves whether the label is a benefit or a burden, and whether it harms us more than it helps us to conceptualize PMS as a medical or psychiatric disorder. Thank you all for your attention."

As soon as these closing words are uttered, the group starts to whisper, and many hands go up.

"I thought we'd wait till the presentations are finished before we open for discussion," Mary Liston says uncertainly, "but I see that's not realistic. Why don't we have a few questions and comments before moving on. Helena, did you want to say something?"

"I certainly do," replies an agitated listener, leaping to her feet. "Those are nice words for a sociologist, someone who hasn't experienced PMS. You have some nerve coming here and telling us there's something wrong with medical treatment. I know I speak for many PMS sufferers when I say that without progesterone therapy I'd be a dead duck. Besides me, several women here are members of PMS Action, a nonprofit organization founded in 1980 whose 'mission is to educate laypersons and professionals about PMS.'[24] For almost twenty years I went from doctor to doctor looking for relief. I suffered fatigue, pains in my joints, backaches, eating binges, and headaches. I was depressed, I got fat, and I worried that I had a serious psychiatric disease. I went to ordinary doctors, gynecologists, psychiatrists, psychologists, osteopaths, and chiropractors. I even had acupuncture. Nothing helped.

"Finally, after I started doing my own research about PMS in the library, 'I discovered "premenstrual syndrome" and the work of Dr. Katharina Dalton. . . . I went to England to see [Dr. Dalton], who diagnosed my complex of symptoms as premenstrual syndrome. Since [then], I have been on progesterone therapy and close to asymptomatic.'[25] Today, along with many other members and supporters of PMS Action, I believe that medical treatment is the only correct approach. We provide counseling to thousands of women, often together with members of their families. And we 'maintain a national listing of physicians who treat women with PMS. In order to receive referrals from PMS Action, a physician must include progesterone therapy as a treatment option.'[26] I'm sorry to say this, Professor Gordon, but you're doing a disservice to women with your abstract notions about the medicalization of PMS."

A small group of women burst into applause as Helena finishes and sits down. "I guess we'll have a few more brief comments," Mary Liston says resignedly. She turns to another member of the audience who raised her hand as soon as Laura Gordon finished speaking. "Dr. Schein, did you have a comment?"

"Yes, I think there are scientific and medical issues that go beyond the scope of tonight's meeting. Professor Gordon was correct when she said there continues to be controversy and uncertainty about the etiology of PMS."

"Could you please use ordinary language at this meeting, Dr. Schein?" Helena interrupts.

"Sorry. 'Etiology' is a technical term for the cause or causes of a disease."

"Thank you."

"Anyway, as I was saying, I think Professor Gordon went a bit too far in rejecting a medical approach to PMS, but she was right when she said the studies of progesterone therapy have been flawed and inconclusive. I've been involved in clinical research on PMS for over ten years now, and I'm very familiar with the scientific literature. 'There are virtually no conclusive data available concerning its diagnosis or measurement, or specifying the precise endocrine and biochemical changes involved; nor are there any reliable studies enabling us to offer adequate treatment to patients.'[27] The theories about progesterone deficiency remain unproven, and the problem with most of the studies to date is that they've lacked placebo controls. You simply can't draw scientifically valid conclusions about whether or not a therapy works without comparing the group receiving the experimental treatment with another group that receives a placebo—I mean, an inactive substance. With PMS, in particular, the placebo effect of any therapy has been shown to be about 40 to 50 percent, and sometimes even more.[28]

"I think it does a disservice to the many women who experience PMS to suggest at a meeting like this that progesterone replacement is *the* answer. 'There are as many studies showing no differences or higher progesterone levels as there are studies showing low progesterone levels in association with the symptoms.' My own hypothesis is that although hormones are certainly involved, 'the problem cannot be as simple as one of progesterone deficiency or increase of estrogen/progesterone ratio.'[29]

"I'm sure everyone here knows that treatments for PMS have included approaches that do not involve any medications, such as yoga, aerobic activity, hypnosis, music therapy, and even masturbation.[30] In addition to hormone treatments, other drugs have been tried—psychotropic medications—and vitamins. As I already mentioned, the placebo effect is generally reported to be 40–50 percent. 'Of all the available treatments, the use of progesterone or progestagens has received the most publicity and almost fanatical support.'[31] I think fanaticism has no place in medical science, and if the purpose of this support group is to benefit women with PMS, it's our obligation to reject bad science."

Helena jumps up again. "Dr. Schein, have you ever had PMS?"

"No, I haven't," Dr. Schein replies.

"Then who are you to talk? First we had a sociologist giving us a bunch of abstract academic claptrap; now we have a doctor spouting medical science about PMS. It really galls me! This is a community support group, not a medical convention. Please take your hypotheses elsewhere, doctor."

"I think it's time to go on to our next speaker," Mary Liston ventures.

"Excuse me, Mary, can't we see where this leads?" queries Laura Gordon.

"All right then, but just a few more comments before we go on. Pardon me for pointing, but I don't know your name—"

The unidentified woman stands up slowly. "I just wanted to add something from my own experience. Once I learned that my emotional symptoms were due to PMS, people began treating me like I was looking for excuses to avoid my responsibilities. At work they accused me of being a hypochondriac. At home my husband said I was trying to avoid housework. Even a psychiatrist I went to said I lacked coping skills.[32] I'm not sure I wasn't better off before I had a name for what was wrong with my life. Except for a few women friends I talked to about it, when I'd say the letters 'PMS' people would look at me funny. It was the old story of blaming the victim."

"I had just the opposite experience," another woman volunteers. "Before I knew what was wrong, people treated me like a nut. I'm not married, but men I've been involved with called me neurotic. I walked around feeling guilty all the time and worried that I'd be out of control at any minute. Once my PMS was diagnosed, I felt relieved. Now that I know the cause of my strong emotions and unpredictable behavior, I can accept them better. Not only that, I can predict when they will happen."

"*You* can accept them better, but what about other people? Do they react better or worse when you tell them you have PMS?" the first unidentified woman asks.

The second replies, "I really can't say. I don't go around advertising the fact."

Mary Liston intervenes. "Okay, it's time to move on to our next speaker. Althea Jefferson has agreed to share with us some of the legal developments involving PMS."

"Yes, thank you for inviting me. I know this situation has come up for only very few women, but there are a number of cases in which PMS has been used as a defense in criminal proceedings in order to mitigate responsibility. I represented two clients using this defense. There have also been civil cases in which PMS has been used as a defense. The results have been mixed.

"The first precedents for a 'PMS defense' were set in British courts. In two cases, women who killed another person were convicted of manslaughter rather than murder on grounds of PMS-diminished responsibility.[33] In the first case, which occurred in 1980, a barmaid named Sandie Craddock stabbed another barmaid three times through the heart. Craddock had forty-five prior convictions, many for unexplainable outbursts of violence. In addition, she had attempted suicide a number of times and had been committed to mental institutions on several occasions. Before the trial, she was examined by Katharina Dalton, the British physician whose work on PMS was mentioned earlier. Dr. Dalton examined the defendant personally and also investigated her history, using official records. She diagnosed Craddock as having severe PMS and began to treat her with huge doses of progesterone. According to reports, the defendant's personality and behavior were markedly altered. She became calm and stable following the progesterone treatment.

"Dr. Dalton's diagnosis convinced the prosecution, which reduced the charge against Craddock to manslaughter. The jury convicted her on this charge, and then the court cited PMS again as a factor to mitigate her sentence. Craddock was put on probation while she continued progesterone treatment. So PMS was used twice in *Regina v. Craddock*: once to reduce the charge from murder to manslaughter, and then to avoid punishment for manslaughter.[34]

"In the second British case, a woman who had no criminal record killed her lover in 1980 by crushing him against a lamppost with her car. Christine English was thirty-seven years old, divorced, with two children. Although she had no criminal record, she had suffered a severe postpartum depression after her second son was born and had attempted suicide. She met her lover, Barry Kitson, in 1976. He was a married alcoholic, and the two fought frequently. Kitson physically abused English during his drinking bouts, following which he would promise to reform—a common pattern in alcohol-induced battering.

"On the day of the killing, Kitson told English he had a date with another woman. After a violent episode in the morning, they had another fight in a pub where English located him. She followed him out of the bar and then drove him around town searching for the other woman. There was more drinking in another pub and more fighting, and Kitson asked English to take him home with her. She refused; there was another fight, and he got out of the car. When he made an obscene gesture at her, she drove the car right at him and smashed him against the lamppost. English immediately was taken to a police station, 'hysterical but clearheaded' and showing remorse. When she left the police station at five o'clock the next morning, she began to menstruate. Kitson died in the hospital two weeks later.

"In the court proceedings, a diagnosis of PMS was used to support a plea of diminished responsibility. Again, Dr. Katharina Dalton testified, along with a psychiatrist, Dr. John Hamilton. These two physicians added a second factor to the plea of diminished responsibility: the likelihood of hypoglycemia, or abnormally low blood sugar. English hadn't eaten for nine hours before she killed Kitson, and the physicians agreed that this may have added to the cause of her actions by inducing hypoglycemia and a reactive surge of adrenalin. The judge accepted the plea of diminished responsibility, finding that the defendant acted under 'wholly exceptional circumstances.' He imposed no sentence but gave English a one-year conditional discharge with a ban on driving.[35]

"Next I'll tell you briefly about the cases I was involved in. In the first, *People v. Santos*, I was the court-appointed attorney for Shirley Santos, a woman from Brooklyn, New York, who in 1981 allegedly beat her four-year-old daughter.[36] Ms. Santos called an ambulance for her daughter after the beating. She was charged with two felonies: second-degree assault, and endangering the welfare of a child. My client said she didn't remember what happened and that she would never hurt her baby. She added that she had just gotten her period. In a pretrial hearing, I argued that PMS, along with fasting that made Ms. Santos hypoglycemic, had caused her to be unconscious of her actions in beating the child.

"The presiding judge found the defense credible and stated that if mental disturbances are admissible evidence, so, too, should physical disturbances be. The prosecutor dropped the felony charge against my client and reduced the guilty plea to harassment, a misdemeanor. The court actually made no authoritative statement about the merits of a PMS defense, but my client was given no sentence, fine, or probation. A separate proceeding in family court, however, resulted in her losing custody of her child.

"The other client I represented was charged with shoplifting.[37] She was a housewife, forty-seven years old, who behaved in a way that showed she was unaware of her situation. Her husband testified that one day each month his wife would obtain inappropriate items from stores. For example, although they had no pets, she would come home with dog food; although their children were grown, she would come home with baby clothes. The husband said his wife could never remember how she got these things. He even kept a diary to try to ensure that she would not have access to the car, cash, or credit cards on the days she was at risk for this behavior. On the basis of the husband's testimony, the charges against my client were dismissed, and she began a successful course of progesterone treatment.

"Other legal cases in which PMS has been used as a defense have involved the crimes of shoplifting, infanticide, arson, forging a prescription, and making false emergency calls.[38] It is obvious that I think PMS can provide a basis for a legal defense. But that doesn't mean it can be used in all cases in which a woman who commits a crime has PMS symptoms. The only circumstances in which PMS can constitute a basis for a legal defense are those in which women experience recurrent, temporary mood disturbance in the premenstrual period, followed by a return to normality afterwards.[39] I think I'll stop here, and answer any questions the audience may have."

Again, many hands go up. Mary Liston calls on a woman who hasn't yet spoken.

"Ms. Jefferson, could you compare PMS with psychosis or other mental conditions used in the insanity defense?"

"That's a tall order," Althea Jefferson replies. "I'll try to summarize briefly. The history of the insanity defense begins in England in 1843 with the M'Naghten case. The M'Naghten test of insanity, still used in many states in America today, focuses on the cognitive aspect of the perpetrator's mental state at the time the crime was committed. Let me see if I can recall the exact wording of the M'Naghten Rules: 'It must be clearly proved that . . . the party accused was laboring under such a defect of reason, from disease of the mind, as not to know the nature and quality of the act he was doing; or, if he did know it, that he did not know he was doing what was wrong.'[40]

"Because the M'Naghten test is purely a cognitive one, many states have added a second criterion for insanity, known as the 'irresistible impulse.'

This test focuses on the lack of voluntariness of the act committed by an accused individual. In other words, the person couldn't keep from doing the act because of an irresistible impulse. Other modifications in the insanity defense were introduced over the years, and as is often the case, today different states have different legal rules regarding insanity. In 1984 the federal government enacted a new insanity law, currently operating in federal jurisdictions, which 'states that a person would not be criminally responsible if, at the time of the commission of the acts, the defendant, as a result of severe mental disease or defect, was unable to appreciate the nature and quality or the wrongfulness of his acts.'[41]

"As I've already said here and in representing my clients, I believe PMS can be used as a legal defense. In fairness, though, I should add that some experts disagree. It is argued that not enough is yet known about PMS to conclude that the condition can be used as the basis for acquittal in criminal behavior. It may, however, be part of a larger mental picture that allows an argument to be made either for insanity, for diminished capacity, or for diminished responsibility.[42] This is a very complex issue in law, with many legal and psychiatric experts disagreeing on many points."

"Let's take one more question before we go on to Andrea Goldwoman's commentary. Yes, please."

Patty Mae Smith stands up hesitantly. "I'm new here tonight, and I'm sorry if this is a stupid question. But are you saying that when a woman who is suffering PMS acts in an abnormal way, she's insane? I mean, even a person who doesn't commit any crime could still behave in ways that aren't normal. Does that mean the woman is crazy? Or insane?"

"Of course not," Ms. Jefferson replies. "In the case of women who do commit crimes during the time when they're having severe PMS symptoms, they aren't fully responsible for their actions. To say that someone isn't fully responsible is not to say that she's crazy."

"That's what I thought. But you've been talking about the insanity defense. Doesn't insanity mean mentally ill?"

"I see why you're confused," Ms. Jefferson responds. "Perhaps it's more like *temporary* insanity. But the main point in the criminal law is to reduce the charge and reduce the sentence for the defendant who suffers from PMS. If you recall, I spoke of 'diminished responsibility.' That's a better way of describing the situation than talking about insanity."

Patty Mae sits down, a puzzled look still on her face. Mary Liston calls on Andrea Goldwoman for her comments.

"I don't really have a specific commentary on the two presentations. But

I want to say a few words about how this whole PMS thing is setting the women's movement back. With heightened public awareness of PMS, fostered by media hype, sexist prejudices are being reinforced. Since all or almost all women menstruate, any woman can be suspected of having PMS and be barred from certain jobs. Any responsible position that requires stability, a high level of skill, or frequent exercise of good judgment might be considered off limits for women. I can hear the arguments now, arguments against women's applying to be airline pilots, seeking to be neurosurgeons, or running for public office. What if a woman starts having PMS symptoms just as she has to land the airplane? or make an incision into the brain? or make a critical decision about international politics? A few years ago there were people who said women couldn't hold responsible jobs because of their 'raging hormones.'[43] Today, they can just substitute the letters PMS.

"If you think I'm exaggerating, just listen to these words from *Time* magazine: 'Days or even two weeks before menstrual bleeding begins, many women experience tenderness and swelling of the breasts, migraine headaches, abdominal bloating and acne. They become lethargic, irritable and depressed. Researchers contend that severely distressed women are apt to have accidents, abuse their children, or commit suicide or violent crime.'[44] Another article that appeared in the *Washington Post* referred to 'the estimated 40% of women who have PMS to one degree or another.'[45] And one in *Harper's Bazaar* stated that 'sociologists have begun to look at the amount of time lost from work because of symptoms apparently related to menstrual periods. . . . And it has been discovered that much time has been lost from work reportedly because of these [symptoms].'[46] Any employer who reads these things will be forced to conclude that refusing to hire women for sensitive positions is good policy, and that maybe discrimination against women in general isn't such a bad idea.

"Further examples show that even the supposedly objective medical literature on PMS contains negative stereotypes of women. An early article by Dr. Dalton and a co-author speaks of women who disturb 'the tranquillity of their homes' every month. 'Guiding their discussion are norms about the "proper" role of adult women. According to these norms, women should have homes with husbands and children living in them, and are responsible for maintaining a happy and harmonious home life.'[47] Granted, Dalton was writing in 1953, before the present phase of the women's movement got started. But this sort of reference to women and home life still persists in the medical literature. An article written in 1981 quotes Dalton's reference to 'a temporary deterioration [in] interpersonal relationships.' 'When they become irritable, tense, or depressed during the premenstrual week,' the authors add, 'marital discord and even baby battering can occur.'[48] These are doctors, writing in 1981, who assume that 'normal' families are happy, and that it is the responsibility of wives and mothers to make sure the happiness of everyone in the family is preserved.

"I think more harm than good is done to women by putting a label like PMS on them. On this point I want to second the remarks made earlier by Laura Gordon. Even in those cases where the PMS label may benefit an individual woman, long-standing negative consequences to her may follow. Labels tend to stick, even when the original grounds for applying them no longer exist. A label creates a stigma, which often outweighs whatever good the label is meant to serve. Still, I acknowledge that a PMS label could benefit some women. My chief objection is the harm it does to women in general. Women as a group are harmed by the social perception that PMS could strike anyone and that you never know when a woman may erupt because of PMS.

"My final comments go to the legal and criminal issues. I'm not an expert on law or psychiatry, but I know enough to say that an insanity plea may be worse for a criminal defendant than a guilty plea. You plead insanity, and if that defense is accepted, you end up in a mental hospital. People have languished there for years. Especially when the disease—if we can call it that—is one that has no cure or effective treatment, as we've heard tonight about PMS, is a mental hospital really a better place to be than a prison? If you plead guilty, there's at least the possibility of a plea bargain, which can reduce the sentence. So a criminal defendant who pleads guilty to the crime might end up in a better place and get out sooner than one who uses the insanity defense.

"Another worry about using PMS as a criminal defense is the potential it raises for screening women to see if they're at risk for severe PMS. Put the biological psychiatrists together with the criminologists, and you've got a dangerous combination. Biological psychiatrists are looking to the chemicals of the body for the root causes of every kind of behavior. Criminologists are ready to pounce on these hypotheses and use them in the service of crime prevention. Listen to this statement by one criminologist of this persuasion: 'In recent years there have been a number of studies relating criminal behavior to genetic processes and neurological and hormonal defects. Some of the disorders discussed in the literature include sociopathy, epilepsy, brain dysfunction, left hemisphere dysfunction, head trauma, alcoholism and drug abuse, hormonal defects (including testosterone defects in males and premenstrual syndrome in females), nutritional and dietary problems, . . . hypoglycemia, and other biochemical disturbances in the brain. Hair analysis can inferentially detect brain damage from lead and cadmium as well as nutritional defects. . . . Some criminal and non-criminal subpopulations have been differentiated as to concentrations of lead, cadmium, iron, sodium, potassium, copper, and zinc in the brain.'[49]

"Now doesn't that boggle the mind? Or should I say the brain? Where do you think this perspective leads? I'll tell you where it leads, by quoting another passage or two from this criminologist in cahoots with biological psychiatry. 'If we are to establish a model which prevents future criminal behavior, we must first deal with the issue of prediction of such future behavior. We are inaccurate in our efforts to predict violence because of our sloppy prediction methods. We use verbal interviews and paper-and-pencil tests. If we used neurological measures, evidence suggests that we would obtain more accurate results.'[50] This criminologist goes on to name a few of these predictive measures that have been used so far: studies of the autonomic nervous system of mentally abnormal offenders, physiological measures of penile responses of sex offenders, and high norepinephrine levels of aggressive individuals.[51]

"So, the next logical step is screening women for PMS in order to prevent crime. Even if the screening is limited to those who have reported some symptoms, that's as many as *half* of all women, as we heard earlier this evening. How many of you in this room would like to be screened for your criminal tendencies, based on your PMS? Don't raise your hands, I already know the answer. Not only would you be screened; you'd also be treated, possibly against your will. I beg your indulgence one last time: here's what the criminologist says. 'Biochemical and neurological tests could be run on our potential offender populations. Hair analysis and PET scans could be used to diagnose potential behavioral problems and pre-delinquency conditions. Drug therapies are available for schizophrenia, depression, sociopathy, and alcoholism. Depo-Provera (an anti-androgen) is being used for the treatment of sex offenders, and progesterone therapy is being used for PMS offenders. Hypoglycemia, hyperactivity, alcoholism, and learning disabilities are among the behavioral disorders which can be treated.'[52]

"I'm sure you can see why I think the PMS label does more harm than good, and why we should resist mightily the argument that women are benefited by a diagnosis of PMS. Organizations like this support group can do a lot more for women in general, as well as for those who experience symptoms of so-called PMS, than the medical-biological-psychiatric-legal-criminological establishment."

"Thank you Andrea. We're now open for general discussion. Helena, did you have a question?"

"Not a question, Mary, a comment. What we've just heard is more ideology. Earlier we heard from a sociologist, telling us what's wrong with medicalization of PMS. Now we're told that PMS is bad for the women's movement. I'm sorry to have to say this, but a women's movement that doesn't care about individual women's suffering is for the birds."

Althea Jefferson adds: "I agree. Different things may benefit different women. A feminist perspective should be able to speak for all women and still recognize individual differences. The idea that doing away with the PMS label will eliminate PMS is ridiculous. Also, I object to these attacks on Katharina Dalton. She has devoted her professional life to helping women with PMS, and she's being portrayed here as some sort of demon."

"Althea, can you respond to Andrea's comments about prison being a better place than a mental hospital for women who commit crimes ·nder the influence of PMS?"

"Well, there may be some truth to that, in certain situations. But those aren't the only two choices when a PMS defense is used in criminal proceedings. In fact, as my experience and that of Katharina Dalton shows, the PMS defense is used to argue for diminished capacity and to mitigate responsibility for the crime. As I said in reply to an earlier question, PMS itself isn't sufficient cause to enter a plea of 'not guilty by reason of insanity.' And there's controversy among psychiatrists over whether PMS should be considered a disease or disorder. So it's not very likely that using PMS as a legal defense will result in a judge sending the woman to an institution for the criminally insane for thirty years."

"Okay," Mary Liston says, "any more questions or comments before we close the formal portion of the meeting? Yes, please—" Mary signals to a woman she doesn't recognize.

"Thank you, I'm new to this community. I'm a social worker, and I just moved from Cleveland, where I was vice-chair of a women's group. We invited guest speakers to a couple of meetings devoted to PMS, as you have done here tonight. We had a psychiatrist from University Hospital, a gynecologist from Case Western Reserve who specializes in treating PMS, and a law professor who spoke about the legal issues. I must say, our meetings in Cleveland were very different from what I've seen this evening. We never had all this name-calling and backstabbing. We all tended to see PMS as a problem for many women but with a variety of possible solutions. The experts shared their knowledge and viewpoints with the laypersons in the audience, and it was a mutually satisfying experience. Frankly, I don't see how anyone can be helped by a meeting where everyone is attacking or being attacked.

"As a feminist, I believe there's room for different approaches to PMS, as well as to other problems women face. Just as not all women are alike, not all feminist perspectives are alike. If I could suggest something, I think this group should have a follow-up meeting without the invited experts. With all due respect to their expertise, we've heard their presentations, and now it's time to discuss the different viewpoints openly, without so much hostility. I'd volunteer to moderate the discussion."

Members of the audience nod and murmur. Mary Liston speaks. "Thank you, and welcome to our group. I'd like to take you up on your suggestion, if everyone agrees." More nods, and a smattering of applause.

"Very well, then, that's less work for me in preparation for our next meeting. Let's adjourn for some refreshments. We have decaf and cider, fresh fruit, and some homemade baked goods prepared without sugar or artificial sweeteners. Thank you all for coming tonight. See you next week."

❧

Patty Mae Smith approaches the table spread with refreshments. She asks one of the women cutting a pan of raisin-nut bars if there's any regular coffee.

"No, we just have decaf here. We try to set a good example for our group members in adhering to dietary recommendations for PMS."

Patty Mae has a glass of cider and two raisin-nut bars. Then she walks out to her car, confused and a little depressed.

CHAPTER 6

Controlling Psychiatric Patients

Mercy Hospital is a 750-bed private, not-for-profit facility. Originally owned and operated by a Catholic religious order, the hospital is now secular, affiliated with the local medical school. The hospital has the staffing shortages common to large inner-city institutions. The two top floors are short-term psychiatric wards, where patients are normally admitted voluntarily but can also be involuntarily committed, usually for no longer than three or four weeks. Patients still in need of hospitalization beyond that time are transferred to a long-term psychiatric facility. Because of the staffing shortage, adequate supervision is not available for all patients on the psychiatric ward.

Frannie Amiga had agreed to enter the hospital voluntarily when she became suicidal after learning about her HIV infection. The psychiatrists there started her on a course of antidepressants and anti-anxiety drugs. She asked the doctors please not to disclose the fact that she was HIV-positive to her brother and sister-in-law.

Two days after being admitted, she calls Larry on the phone. "Hi Larry, I'm here."

"Fran! how're you doing? You okay?"

"Yeah, I guess so. You know, I felt real bad about not being able to do the surrogacy thing for you."

"Fran, I'm sorry. Bonnie and I are really sorry. We should never have asked you."

"It's not your fault, Larry. Just get that idea out of your head, okay? I really wanted to help you guys."

"Do you want us to visit? Do you need anything?"

"No, I'll be out of here in a few days. But there is one thing you can do for me, Lar. Remember that guy I used to go out with, Vinnie Martino? Could you find out for me where he is these days?"

"I'll try, but how come? I thought you had a big fight with that guy when you broke up."

"I just want to know where he is. Please, don't ask questions. Just do me the favor, will you?"

"Sure, Fran, I'll see what I can find out. Call us any time. And if you want company, just let us know."

❧

Frannie shares a two-person room with a middle-aged woman suffering from severe depression. She never initiates a conversation herself and only mumbles a word or two in response to Frannie's attempts. Frannie overhears two psychiatrists discussing the possibility of administering electroconvulsive therapy to her roommate, who has not responded to several different medications. "I thought they gave up that barbaric stuff," Frannie says to herself. "I wonder what they have in mind for me."

Frannie undergoes brief evaluation sessions each day with a psychiatrist and has longer daily meetings with a psychiatric social worker. She declines to participate in the group therapy meetings on the ward. After seven days Frannie decides she's had enough of the hospital and tells the psychiatrist assigned to her that she wants to leave.

Frannie's psychiatrist is Joshua Gold, in his last year of the residency training program. Soft-spoken and gentle, Dr. Gold says, "Ms. Amiga, you've shown very positive improvement in the week you've been here. But we think you could benefit from another week under our supervision."

"I'd like to leave, Dr. Gold. I've had enough of this place. As you said yourself, I'm better now. I never think about killing myself anymore. I want to live life to the fullest, now that I know I may not have too much longer. I can't live my life to the fullest in this place."

"I agree, you're not suicidal any more. But another week of supervision is advisable."

"What do you mean by 'supervision'?" What are you supervising me for? Remember, I signed myself in here voluntarily."

"To be honest, Ms. Amiga, we're a bit worried about the hostility you've been expressing. Especially toward your former lover. We want to hear more about the man you hold responsible, so we can help you process your feelings. We understand your anger, but we don't want you to act on it. It's important that you talk more about your feelings."

Frannie's eyes flash. "Wouldn't any sane person want to get revenge? That guy gave me AIDS! Wait'll I get my hands on him—"

Joshua Gold tells Frannie he'll consult with his colleagues and speak with her tomorrow. Later that day he asks Blanche Williams, the social worker, and Dr. Diaz, the attending psychiatrist, if they have time for a brief consultation about Frannie. Shortly after 5:00 P.M. the three convene in Dr. Diaz's office. Dr. Gold begins.

"I wanted to consult about Frannie Amiga, the patient in 904B with HIV infection. She's been here a week and no longer appears to have suicidal ideation. Now she's asked to be discharged, but I don't think she's ready yet. Frankly, I'm worried about her potential for acting out. In our daily sessions she refers repeatedly to 'the guy who gave me AIDS.' I'm afraid she could really do something to him when she leaves the hospital. What do you think?"

Blanche Williams speaks up. "I tend to agree. I've actually heard her say on more than one occasion, 'I'll kill the guy who gave me AIDS.' She hasn't mentioned his name to me, though."

Dr. Diaz pauses before speaking. "I don't know this patient, so I can't make a clinical judgment at this point, but you know, of course, that her reactions are perfectly natural for someone who learns about a fatal condition. She may be stuck at the angry stage; she may need time to reach acceptance."

"But this patient never exhibited the denial we get with cancer patients," Dr. Gold observes.

"I'm not sure these stages are always invariant," Dr. Diaz replies. "But tell me more about her anger. Does she appear to be angry at everyone? Or just the boyfriend?"

"She's focused on the former lover," Ms. Williams says. "And she's said more than once that she wants to kill him. That's the part Josh and I are concerned about."

"People often use those words without meaning them," Dr. Diaz responds. "We need more to go on, especially if we're going to try to keep her here against her will. As you know, we psychiatrists aren't very good at predicting dangerousness. And we're on shaky legal ground if we haven't got a sound basis for detaining her."

"Yes, but aren't we on equally dangerous ground if we discharge her and then she goes out and harms someone?" Joshua Gold asks.

"You're referring to Tarasoff?" Dr. Diaz asks.

"You bet!" Joshua retorts.

"Isn't that the case that imposes a 'duty to warn' on psychotherapists?" Blanche Williams asks. "I believe it applies to social workers, as well, when they're doing psychotherapy. We were talking about it at our last staff meeting, but we were not exactly sure what our obligations were according to that case. Dr. Diaz, could you please go over it?"

"I'll try. But remember, the Tarasoff ruling was in California, so strictly speaking, the legal precedent doesn't apply in this state. Anyway, about the case.

"Tatiana Tarasoff was a student at the University of California at Berkeley. She was killed by another student, named Poddar, who met her in a folk-dancing class and fell in love with her. Tarasoff rebuffed Poddar, and he went into a severe depression. After six months he sought help at the university health service. He was treated by a clinical psychologist, who found him 'a danger to the welfare of other people and himself' after he disclosed his intention to kill Tarasoff when she returned from Brazil, where she was spending the summer. Now the therapist didn't warn Tarasoff, but he did contact the campus police. The police detained Poddar, but when he appeared rational and promised them he would stay away from Tarasoff, he was released. Two months later Tarasoff returned from Brazil, and Poddar killed her with a butcher knife.

"As I said, the psychotherapist did do something, but he didn't warn the victim or her parents. The parents brought a wrongful death action against the Board of Regents of the State of California, the campus police, the psychologist who had been involved in Poddar's treatment, and also the psychologist's superior at the clinic, who had said no further action should be taken. The Tarasoff case is usually described in terms of the 'duty to warn,' but the California Supreme Court ruling also mentioned the duty to take other preventive steps if there's reason to believe another person is in danger from the therapist's patient."[1]

"That's a heavy burden!" Ms. Williams exclaims. "How can a therapist know, if a patient threatens to harm someone, when it's appropriate to betray confidentiality?"

"There was a mild uproar in the psychiatric community after the case was publicized," Dr. Diaz continues. "Confidentiality, of course, has an important role in a therapeutic relationship. One of the judges who dissented from the majority in the Tarasoff case made that point. He cited three reasons why assurance of confidentiality is especially important for psychiatric treatment. The first is that without that assurance, people who need psychiatric help would be deterred from seeking treatment. Second, the guarantee of confidentiality is essential if psychiatric patients are to make the full disclosures that may be necessary for effective treatment. The third reason goes back to the success of the therapy itself—the importance of maintaining the patient's trust in his psychiatrist.[2] I think the judge was right on all three counts."

"What concerns me in this case is, how do we decide whether this patient is dangerous?" Dr. Gold says. "We know there's no real basis for making such predictions, except when we know the patient has committed acts of violence in the past."

"I agree," replies Dr. Diaz, "and so did one of the dissenting justices. He criticized the majority for relying on the 'standard of care' in this area of psychiatry and cited articles in the professional literature which argue that in the psychiatric field, therapists cannot accurately predict dangerousness. This means that the standard of care fails to provide a relevant criterion for judging a therapist's decision."

"This is useful, but how does it apply to our patient in 904B?" Joshua Gold asks.

"I'd like to talk with the patient myself," Dr. Diaz answers. "But from what I've heard from both of you, I have my doubts that a prediction of dangerousness is justified. She has no history of violent behavior, and she's reacting somewhat appropriately to a piece of very bad news."

"I don't doubt your psychiatric judgment, but what about our liability? We could all get sued up the kazoo if we discharge this patient and she goes out and stabs the guy. We have to protect ourselves, don't we?" young Dr. Gold questions his superior.

"That's a consideration," Dr. Diaz replies, "but not the main one. Our first obligation is to our patients. The second, when it arises, is to prevent harm from befalling innocent parties at the hands of our patients. Only after these obligations are met should we begin considering the issue of our potential liability."

"That's a nice ideal. I don't know about you, but I have to live in the real world," Dr. Gold declares.

"I'll arrange to speak with the patient myself tomorrow," Dr. Diaz says. "Then we can confer again."

The next morning, Dr. Diaz interviews Frannie Amiga. The psychiatrist is surprised at the depth of Frannie's anger and decides that caution is warranted. When Frannie threatens to walk out of Mercy Hospital, the psychiatrist urges her to cooperate, saying they will evaluate her readiness to leave after the weekend. Dr. Diaz notifies the administrator on duty that a patient on the psychiatric floor has threatened to leave the hospital and asks that a security guard be stationed near the elevators over the weekend.

❁

On Monday morning, Dr. Diaz is in her office reading her morning mail when Joshua Gold bursts in. "Marta, I need your help. Remember the patient we talked about last week? The HIV-infected woman who's threatening to kill her former boyfriend? Well, listen to this. At morning rounds, one of the nurses said that Ms. Amiga was reported to be having sex with two other patients on the ward."

"Are they sure about that?" Dr. Diaz asks.

"As sure as they ever are. We know it goes on, and there's little we can do about it."

"I know, but now we have a much bigger problem on our hands. I think we should call a special staff meeting to discuss this matter."

The next day at noon, psychiatrists, nurses, and social workers, all carrying bag lunches or carry-out containers, troop into the small conference room on the ninth floor of the hospital. Dr. Diaz addresses the group as everyone gets settled.

"I'd like to get started right away. Donna, could you please close the door. Thank you. As many of you already know, a dilemma has come up. A patient on the ward who we know is HIV-positive has had sexual encounters with other patients. Let's get the facts before we discuss what steps to take. Can any of you provide me with information?"

One of the nurses raises her hand. "I'm the one who reported the incident to Dr. Gold. When I came in for the morning shift, the patient in 904B wasn't in her bed. I didn't think anything of it until I went into 908. I knew something was up when I saw a woman sleeping in the bed, because 908 is shared by two male patients. I recognized the woman as the patient from 904. She didn't have anything on."

"Where was the patient whose bed she was in?"

"I didn't know where he was. But the other patient in 908 was there. When he saw me looking at the woman in the other bed, he grinned. He said Hector had gone out to have a cigarette. This patient—his name is Mustafa—told me that sometime after midnight Hector told him, Mustafa, to take a walk for a little while. Mustafa said he refused. Hector went out of the room and came back with Ms. Amiga. Mustafa said he watched them doing it."

"What did you do next?" Dr. Diaz asks.

"I went out and got a hospital robe. Then I went back to 908 and woke Ms. Amiga, gave her the robe, and told her to get back to her room. As she was leaving, she winked at Mustafa."

Dr. Diaz looks around the room. "Does anyone have anything to add?"

The nurse named Donna speaks up. "When I came on my shift Sunday morning, the night nurse told me there was hanky-panky going on. She said Mustafa was in 904, in bed with the woman patient in bed B."

"Why didn't you report this?"

"Well, to be honest, I didn't want to get the night nurses in trouble."

"We have to know about these things," Marta Diaz admonishes. "I know we're understaffed, but we must have better supervision of these patients."

A junior resident blurts out, "We don't really have to worry about sexual exploitation in this case, do we? After all, this is a woman patient seducing men."

"That's a sexist remark if I ever heard one, Gary," a social worker says. "We have to protect all our patients from sexual exploitation. They're all vulnerable."

"Come on," Gary replies. "These guys are just doing in here what they'd be doing on the street. What do you think, they're virgins?"

The social worker becomes agitated. "That's not the point. They're in the hospital, and they're psychiatric patients. Hector Valenzuela is here because he went out of control after a two-day binge on crack cocaine, and Mustafa Moore is schizophrenic."

A nurse sitting at the side of the room raises her hand timidly.

"There's another patient," Sheila volunteers.

"What do you mean?"

"I mean, I saw Ms. Amiga with another male patient."

"When was this?"

"Friday afternoon, just before I went off my shift."

"Good God!" Joshua Gold exclaims. "That was just after we told her we weren't going to discharge her."

"Sounds like she was acting out. Who was the male patient, Sheila?" Dr. Diaz asks.

"Mr. Erlbaum."

"Billy Erlbaum? He's only eighteen! And he's so impaired I can't believe he'd know what to do," the resident named Gary pipes up.

"His parents had him committed after he sexually assaulted his younger sister," Blanche Williams says. "He may have impaired thinking, but he's not asexual. We're trying to arrange placement for him now."

"So, that makes three patients Ms. Amiga has had sex with."

"Three we know about," Gary says.

"Our time is running out," Marta Diaz warns. "Let's have some recommendations. We can't allow the situation to continue."

"What are our options?" Joshua Gold asks. "Ideally, we should have better supervision of these patients, but we know that's not going to happen."

"Why not put the promiscuous lady in isolation?" Gary asks.

"We can't do that," Dr. Diaz states. "She doesn't meet the criteria for such an extreme measure."

"Why is it extreme? She's putting other patients at risk, isn't she?"

"The law doesn't allow us to lock up psychiatric patients except in case of emergency or imminent danger to others."

"I think there's imminent danger when she can pass on a lethal disease! It's the same as if she came at other patients with a knife."

"It's not the same at all. If she came at them with a knife, there would be a clear intent to harm them. In the case of sexual acts, a person is just seeking gratification."

"What if a patient gets gratification out of stabbing other people? Would that excuse the behavior because his intent isn't to do harm?"

"Hold on, this patient isn't behaving in this way because she's seeking sexual gratification. She's acting out, because she thinks her former lover gave her AIDS—"

"We're getting off the track," Dr. Diaz interrupts the animated chatter. "Isolation is out of the question, at least until we get some legal advice. I'd like to hear what you think of disclosing to the men who had sex with Ms. Amiga that they've been exposed to HIV infection."

"What would be the point?" Donna asks.

"State law permits physicians to disclose to regular sex partners or needle sharers of an infected person that they have been exposed to the virus."

"Then what?"

"Well, for one thing, those who have been exposed can take steps to avoid passing the infection on to others."

"Does that make any sense here in the psych ward?"

"Obviously, it does. As you can see, patients are having sex with each other."

"Yeah, but this is a psych ward. Just look at the patients. One of her partners is an out-of-control crack addict, another is schizophrenic, and the third is totally out of it. What good would it do to give a verbal warning to these men? Let's be realistic, guys," Gary insists.

Joshua Gold speaks up. "It seems to me there are two different concerns here. One is to try to prevent further spread of AIDS. The other is the question of whether these men have a right to know they may have been infected. And we mustn't forget, they may not have been infected. One or two sexual encounters with an infected person doesn't necessarily spread the virus."

"There's a third concern, Josh," Dr. Diaz points out. "We can't overlook our obligation to our patients to preserve confidentiality. That has to be factored in somehow. The state law that permits disclosure to a partner also prohibits revealing the name of the infected person. All you're supposed to say is, 'Someone who has HIV infection has named you as a sex partner or needle sharer.' "

A nurse raises her hand. "Wouldn't it simplify things if we knew whether any of these men already have HIV infection? I mean, if a person is already infected, what's the point of telling them they've been exposed again?"

"That may be true for them, but there are still the other patients to consider. If we let this loose cannon stay on the wards, she could be in bed with every man on the floor."

"Wait, you're all overlooking an obvious point. If we tell any of these guys they've been exposed to the AIDS virus, they'll know who the infected person is, even if we don't tell them her name; they don't have to be wizards in logic to figure it out. Then they'll tell everyone else on the ward."

"I'm not sure what point you're making. Are you saying it would be impossible to preserve confidentiality?"

"Yes, but there's another, more important point. Once everyone knows that Ms. Amiga is HIV-positive, no one else will go near her."

"Maybe, maybe not."

"Someone may go near her—with the intention of stabbing her to death. It's happened, you know."

"That would be self-defeating. The stabber puts himself at greater risk from all the blood—probably even at greater risk than from sexual contact."

Dr. Diaz interrupts once again. "Let's explore the suggestion made a moment ago that we try to determine whether any of these men is already infected with the virus. What do you think?"

Joshua Gold speaks first. "We'll have to inform anyone who tests positive that they're infected, and they'll need to be counseled before and after the test. Besides, we'll have to get their consent to test their blood for HIV antibodies. What reason will we give them? And what if they lack the capacity to consent? Or what if they refuse? We have to think these things through before we act."

Gary responds, "Aw, come on. These are psych patients. We have to protect ourselves and the hospital. Let's find out the score first, then deal with these problems later. We can just draw the blood, say it's for some lab tests. These guys won't ask questions. We're the doctors. If things don't work out right, no one will put too much stock in the word of a mental patient anyway."

"We have to stick to our ethics," Dr. Diaz insists. "And there are legal constraints, as well. Psychiatric patients have rights, and so do AIDS patients. In this state it's against the law to test anyone's blood for HIV without consent. The law also requires pretest counseling, as well as post-test counseling for those found to be seropositive. I think we should find out first whether these three patients have the capacity to grant informed consent for the HIV test; if they do, then we ask their permission to find out their HIV status."

Most of the staff nod in agreement. Gary and the nurse who first suggested that the patients be tested are whispering to each other, apparently unhappy with the plan.

Joshua Gold and another senior psychiatry resident interview Hector Valenzuela, Mustafa Moore, and Billy Erlbaum to evaluate their capacity to grant informed consent. The psychiatrists on the staff have been properly trained not to assume that a diagnosis of mental illness renders a patient incapable of understanding the information necessary for granting informed consent. The young psychiatrists conclude that Mustafa and Hector have the capacity to consent, but that Billy Erlbaum is too cognitively impaired to understand the necessary information. Mustafa and Hector consent to the blood test. The doctors learn from Erlbaum's chart that his parents were appointed his legal guardians when he turned eighteen, so they are asked to consent to the HIV blood test for their son. They agree.

The patients are counseled by specially trained personnel from the hospital's AIDS team. An initial test called "ELISA" and a confirmatory test ("Western Blot") are performed, and in a week the results come back to the hospital. Billy Erlbaum's and Mustafa Moore's test results are negative but Hector Valenzuela's blood is found to be HIV-positive. For the post-test counseling session with Hector, both the trained AIDS counselor and Dr. Joshua Gold are present.

"Good morning, Hector," Dr. Gold greets the patient.

"Mornin'," the patient replies.

"Hector, we have to talk to you about something. This is Ms. Brown, a counselor in the hospital. Okay?"

"Okay."

Ms. Brown begins. "Hector, you remember we asked you a couple of weeks ago if we could draw some blood?"

"Yeah, I 'member."

"Do you remember what it was for? Why we wanted to test your blood?"

"Mmmm, yeah. I 'member."

"Could you tell us now what you remember?"

"You were talkin' 'bout AIDS. You said you wanna test my blood for AIDS. I said okay."

"That's right, Hector. Well, the tests have come back. Hector, we're very sorry to have to tell you this. Your blood tests positive for the AIDS virus. Now that doesn't mean—"

"What d'ya mean, 'tests positive'? What do you sayin'? I tol' you I don' use needles! I smoke crack and weed. No needles, you hear what I say? Is wrong. Is a mistake. The test is wrong."

"Hector, I think we explained to you that the test is done twice. Then the blood is tested again by a different method. I think we have to believe the test results."

"I don' believe. You can believe."

Ms. Brown speaks softly. "Hector, it's not only needles that pass on AIDS from one person to another. Remember, when we spoke to you before we told you that sexual behavior can also spread AIDS. Remember?"

"Yeah, I 'member. But I tol' you then, an' I tell you again, I'm not a homo! You accuse me of bein' a homo, I gonna sue you! You can't call me a homo 'cause this test comes back and says I have AIDS! I never had sex with no men!"

Josh reassures the patient. "We believe you, Hector. But the virus is also spread through sex between men and women. It's more common for women to get it from men than for men to get it from women. But both are possible."

"I don' believe it."

"Hector, when you were selling crack, did you go into crack houses?"

"Sure."

"What was going on in there?"

"What d'you think? Lotsa people. Girls. Men. Smoking crack, having sex. Some girls in the crack house, they don' have no money, but they give sex for crack." He paused and smiled. "I got lotsa sex from those girls."

"Hector, we have your hospital chart from when you last came in for treatment. You were at the STD clinic, weren't you?

"Huh?"

"Were you treated here at the clinic for a sexually transmitted disease? Venereal disease? Clap? Herpes?"

"Oh, yeah, yeah. I had some sores down there."

"Well, that may explain how you picked up the AIDS virus. You can't be sure that the girls you had sex with in the crack house weren't infected with AIDS, can you?"

"How could I know it? They don' wear no sign sayin' 'I'm clean' or 'I'm dirty.'"

"Hector, your blood tests positive for the AIDS virus, but you're not sick. It could be a very long time before you have any clinical symptoms, I mean, before you start feeling sick. The thing is to take good care of yourself now. When you have HIV infection, you may get sick more easily with other things. Your body can't fight infections as well as it should."

"What difference it gonna make now? I have AIDS, I'm gonna die from it. Not right now, maybe, but later. When I get outa this hospital, I'm jus' gonna have a good time."

"You wouldn't want to spread the disease to others, would you? Part of our counseling here is to educate patients who are infected to try not to infect others. We'd like to tell you just how to—"

"You jus' tol' me I got AIDS from the others. Where you think I go when I leave here? Back home. Back to the street. Prob'ly back to the crack house. You say I get it from those girls, right? So how I'm gonna give it back to them? They already got it, no?"

As Ms. Brown has learned from experience, posttest counseling often requires more than one session. She says, "Hector, we'll come back and talk with you again tomorrow. Meanwhile, if you have any questions, if there's anything you'd like to ask me or Dr. Gold, please call for either one of us. Okay?"

"Okay."

"We'll see you tomorrow, Hector," Joshua Gold adds.

Outside the room, Josh asks Ms. Brown: "Is there any reason to tell Hector that his sexual partner here in the hospital is HIV-positive?"

"Absolutely not. You know he couldn't have acquired it from her; sero-conversion doesn't occur that fast. He was infected before he came here, so that relieves us of any obligation to disclose that he's been exposed to someone who is infected."

"What about the other two patients? The ones whose tests came back negative?"

"I have to think about that. You know, in the other areas of this hospital, sexual encounters between patients are very rare. This is not a problem that we normally have to deal with on the AIDS unit."

"We may have some obligation to them. I'll tell Dr. Diaz about the test results and the counseling session with Hector. I'll get back to you."

After Joshua speaks with Dr. Diaz, she decides to ask for advice from the hospital's ethics committee. The topic is put on the agenda of the next monthly meeting. In anticipation, Dr. Gold and Dr. Diaz prepare brief oral presentations for the committee and call on a colleague with expertise in forensic psychiatry to join them at the meeting.

❧

At 4:30 P.M. on the first Tuesday of the month, members of the ethics committee crowd into a small conference room the the third floor of Mercy Hospital. The committee chairman is Dr. Ira Becker, a professor of medicine at the medical school. The committee comprises physicians from several other departments, three nurses and two social workers from the hospital, a chief resident, a medical student, a hospital administrator, a professor from the university's law school faculty, and the bioethicist Teddi Chernacoff.

Joshua Gold starts by recounting the incidents that have taken place on the inpatient psychiatric floor, the fact that Frannie Amiga is HIV-positive, the counseling and testing of the other patients, and the session with Hector Valenzuela. He sums up the ethical issues raised by the entire situation:

"First, we have a psychiatric patient who we believe poses a threat to a particular individual outside the hospital, but we are uncertain just how great a threat of harm is involved. So the first ethical dilemma is the conflict between the need to prevent harm to innocent parties, and the obligation to respect the liberty of someone who hasn't committed any crime. This patient has been heard to say, 'I'll kill the guy who gave me AIDS,' but to be honest, we don't have the ability to tell whether she'll carry out her threat. Psychiatry does have areas of expertise, but making predictions of dangerousness isn't one of them.

"The second ethical dilemma relates to the patient's sexual behavior on the wards. She's had sex with three other patients, and we've determined that one was already HIV-positive. But what about the other two? Should they be told that they've been exposed to the AIDS virus? Or do we have a higher obligation to preserve the confidentiality of a patient? And what can we do—ethically and legally—to prevent further sexual encounters on the wards?"

"Wow, that's a barn-burner," a physician exclaims. "On our service, we only have to deal with simple ethical problems like when to pull the plug."

Another committee member blurts out: "You're dealing with life and death in this case, too. I really don't see how the ethics of protecting patient confidentiality can compete with the duty to preserve life."

"We're dealing with probabilities here. There's only a probability, not a certainty, that this patient will go out and try to kill her former lover. It's the same with the sex and AIDS thing. It's possible, but not at all likely, that people who have sex on one or two occasions will transmit the virus. It's not so easy to resolve an ethical dilemma when we're working in probabilities."

"How high does the probability of harm have to be before we can detain a person involuntarily? Is there any standard in psychiatry?"

"Not really," Marta Diaz replies. "We don't even have the tools to assess the probability in a precise manner."

"This isn't a psychiatric question; it's a legal matter," the hospital administrator asserts. "Isn't that right, Evan?" he turns to the lawyer on the committee.

"It's both. As in many other areas, the law doesn't speak clearly on this issue. There are no statutes; all we have are some court opinions, and not even those in this jurisdiction."

"So how can we know what the law is?"

Evan replies, "The best we can do is try to predict what the courts will do if a case comes before them."

"That's not very comforting to me," the administrator says. "We have to protect the hospital, you know."

Dr. Becker intervenes. "I think we should approach the case and the issues it raises systematically. We have several different issues before us, and it would be best to take them in turn. Can we start with the problem of sexual activity on the psychiatric ward? That seems to be the most pressing problem, and one for which we need to seek an immediate solution. Dr. Gold, can you tell us more about that?"

"Dr. Diaz is going to talk about that to the committee. We've each prepared a brief presentation, and this is her topic," Joshua says.

Marta Diaz stands to address the group. "Sexual contact between patients is generally prohibited on inpatient psychiatric units. But it goes on anyway, in other hospitals as well as here. From an ethical point of view, the staff makes the assumption that sex on the wards is not in the best interest of psychiatric patients. The basis for that position is rarely stated clearly; however, I can give three reasons why hospitals and staff support the prohibition.

"The first is based on what I call a moralistic stance: sex between casual acquaintances is wrong and should not be allowed in a health facility. The second expresses a legal worry: hospital staff and administration are afraid of potential liability, and a patient who has had a sexual encounter might bring a lawsuit against the hospital.

"The third reason relates to a genuine ethical concern, in my opinion. Patients are vulnerable, whether they are physically or mentally ill, and a hospital has an obligation to protect them from exploitation and harm. Among the potential harms are risk of pregnancy, risk of venereal disease, and the possible harmful effect on the condition that prompted the patient's hospitalization in the first place.[3]

"In many hospitals, all three motives are probably at work, and there may be additional grounds for disallowing sex between patients. But I feel it's important to distinguish ethical reasons from the others, and only the third of those I just stated sounds to me like an ethical basis for the prohibition: vulnerable people stand in need of protection against harm or exploitation. A psychiatric ward, where these vulnerable people are housed, has an obligation to take appropriate steps to ensure their protection.

"When this problem came up, I did a quick review of the literature. One article states that 'within many of the larger facilities, it is not possible to monitor sexual behavior without introducing draconian procedures, which would probably be ineffective and would undermine the therapeutic milieu.'[4] The ineffectiveness of such procedures alone would be sufficient argument against using them, from both an ethical and a practical standpoint. When we add the prospect of invading patients' privacy and

imposing coercive measures, it becomes ethically unacceptable to introduce vigilant monitoring of the sexual behavior of inpatients. That's my
opinion, at least.

"In my reading I did come across another viewpoint about the appropriateness of sex among mentally disabled patients that I'd like to share
with you. This is the view that persons with mental disabilities have a right
to sexual expression. The authors note that misinformation, and incorrect
beliefs have persisted in institutional settings. 'These myths include beliefs
that persons with mental disabilities are oversexed, [are] undersexed, lack
control, have diminished cognitive capacity to understand sexual behavior, are unable to make informed decisions regarding sexual partners, are
unable to use contraceptives, and are unable to be parents.'[5] Although the
article I read pertained to mentally retarded and developmentally disabled
individuals rather than to those with psychiatric disorders, similar beliefs
exist regarding mentally ill persons. I think it's consistent to grant people
with mental disabilities or disorders the right to sexual expression and, at
the same time, seek to protect vulnerable individuals. With the spread of
AIDS, we have an ethical obligation to protect even those patients who are
not vulnerable because of a psychiatric disability.

"So, we're faced with the question, how far can we go to protect patients
from the possibility of being exposed to the AIDS virus? There are legal
as well as ethical implications in this situation. As you know, the treatment of mental patients is governed by laws and regulations. My colleague,
Dr. Gupta, works in the area of forensic psychiatry, and I think she can
add a few words about the law."

Dr. Gupta takes up the discussion: "I didn't prepare a formal speech,"
she says. "I'm here mainly as a resource person. But I can tell you that we're
quite limited in the ways we are permitted to treat psychiatric patients.
Laws and regulations have been put in place over the past few decades in response to earlier abuses. For example, court decisions and state regulations
have established patients' right to treatment in order to protect them from
indefinite 'warehousing,' a practice that went on for many years. Courts
have also granted patients a right to refuse treatment, including psychotropic medication that could relieve symptoms, except in an emergency where
without the medication an agitated patient is likely to do immediate harm
to others.

"The laws most relevant to the issue of controlling the sexual behavior
of psychiatric inpatients are those that mandate using the 'least restrictive
alternative.' That requirement probably makes it legally impermissible to
put patients in isolation. One authority, writing about sexual behavior in

the hospital, has said that 'isolation or seclusion in these cases will often seem inappropriate or may be precluded by state regulations.'[6] This is one of the states in which isolation is precluded as a general response to sexual activity among patients. Whether the fact that a patient is HIV-infected would constitute an exception, I just don't know. It has never been tested, so there's no way of knowing how a judge might rule."

"That really leaves things up in the air, doesn't it?" Ira Becker muses. He looks from one psychiatrist to the other. "What about Tarasoff? Does that apply to this situation?"

Dr. Gupta replies: "It certainly applies to the situation of discharging the patient who may be a threat to her former boyfriend, the one she says gave her AIDS. The two situations are parallel, since both involve one person revealing to a therapist an intention to harm another person. Of course, the therapist still has to evaluate the patient's statement and try to determine whether she is speaking seriously and truthfully. But our patient definitely presents us with a Tarasoff-like situation."

"I say, keep her here as long as you can!" the hospital administrator exclaims. "And if you're forced by the law, or by advocacy groups for mental patients, to let her go, then warn the boyfriend, tell the police, and anyone else who should be informed."

"Not so fast, Bob," Dr. Becker says. "We'll get to the hospital's concerns in a bit. I don't think Dr. Gupta has finished—"

"No, I haven't. I was going to go on to discuss whether Tarasoff applies to the situation of an HIV-infected person having sex with other patients. In one respect, it may: the California court 'based its decision in part on its reading of earlier cases holding physicians liable for failing to inform family members of the infectious nature of a patient's condition.'[7] The original precedents for the duty to warn were cases in which the dangerous persons were those who had infectious diseases, rather than those likely to harm others by violent behavior.

"But there's another respect in which Tarasoff may *not* be applicable to our case, and that has to do with the fact that these are seriously impaired psychiatric patients. We need to ask several questions about how similar such patients are to other people about whom a warning would be appropriate. First, there are questions relating to impaired cognition or judgment. Is the patient able to understand the consequences of a given sort of behavior? Does the patient manifest impaired ability to think, reason, or judge, or lack the capacity to control his or her behavior, so that other people are placed at greater risk than they might be from an unimpaired individual? Second, there is the question of whether the patient is able to respond appropriately to a threat of disclosure of sensitive information by bringing his or her behavior under control.

"I would be the last to argue that all psychiatric patients, by definition, are incapable of understanding or unable to control their behavior. These situations call for clinical judgments, which have to be made on a case-by-case basis. If we relied on the Tarasoff duty to warn, we would have to assume that issuing a verbal warning to patients at risk would be sufficient to protect them. But some of our psychiatric patients may fail to comprehend the warning; some may choose not to act appropriately even given the warning; and others may actually experience a worsening of their psychiatric disorder.

"I know you're looking for answers, but we all have to recognize the limits of psychiatry and also the legal uncertainties. On the basis of my experience in both areas, I've told you as much as I can."

"Dr. Becker, can we get to the question of whether the two men who had sex with this infected patient should be informed?" a committee member asks.

"Do you want to deal with that next?" Dr. Becker asks the group. Heads nod affirmatively. "Okay, Evan, could you say a few words about what the law in this state says about disclosure of HIV information?"

"I'd be glad to. Our state has enacted legislation, similar to that in other states, which tries to do two things at once: protect the health of the public, and safeguard the rights of individuals with HIV infection. The law aims to establish strict confidentiality protections for HIV-infected persons yet permit limited disclosure to persons or agencies described as having a 'need to know.' A physician may disclose confidential HIV-related information to the spouse or known sex partner of a person with AIDS or HIV infection. A physician may also disclose such information to persons who are known to have shared needles and syringes with the patient. I guess doctors hoping for clear guidance will be disappointed in this law, since it doesn't *mandate* disclosure to a sexual partner or needle-sharer but, instead, *permits* the doctor to disclose. The law doesn't impose an absolute obligation either to disclose information or to preserve confidentiality. But it does have stiff penalties for disclosure to individuals or agencies who aren't authorized to receive it, such as a patient's employer.

"Doctors will be happy to learn that they are immune from liability whether they disclose or fail to disclose HIV information to a spouse or sexual partner. By the way, the law does say that the doctor may not disclose the name of the infected person, only that an infected person has named the other person as a sexual contact or needle-sharing partner. Finally, a physician put in this situation doesn't have to do the disclosing himself but may inform the health department, and a public health official will contact the person named as a partner of the infected individual."

"What's the point of having a law if it doesn't tell you what you must or must not do?" a physician member of the committee asks.

"Law is like ethics in that respect," Teddi Chernacoff volunteers. "Duties and obligations fall into three categories: actions that are obligatory; actions that are prohibited; and actions that are permitted. Of the three, the third allows for the widest discretion."

"Can we go back to the point of this meeting?" Ira Becker pleads. "We're a long way from reaching closure on any of the issues."

"I don't think we're all that far from deciding what's the right thing to do about the HIV-infected psychiatric patient's discharge," Joshua Gold said. "We're still within the legal limit of how long she can be held here, and given the evaluation of two psychiatrists and the psychiatric social worker, she appears to present a danger to others—one other person, in particular. We'll continue to evaluate her on a daily basis. If we find no improvement, we may have no choice but to seek involuntary commitment to a long-term psychiatric facility."

"That's like imprisoning her," the medical resident objects. "Is it right to commit a basically sane person to a psychiatric institution full of grossly impaired psychiatric patients? I think it's an abuse of psychiatrists' power to do that."

"Would you rather see a homicidal maniac walking the streets?" a nurse asks.

"This patient is certainly not a homicidal maniac," Dr. Diaz affirms. "But at this point, we think she may harm an identifiable person if we discharge her now. In my judgment, this anger is likely to diminish, then disappear. The patient will probably begin to focus more on her HIV infection and her general life prospects than on her desire for revenge on the man who infected her."

"But what if you're wrong about the prognosis?" the medical resident persists. "How can you hold someone indefinitely in a psychiatric hospital? That's a violation of her civil liberties. In a free country you may incarcerate someone only when they've committed a crime. Anything else is preventive detention. That's what they do in totalitarian societies."

"I didn't know you were some kind of radical libertarian," Dr. Becker quips.

"Actually," Teddi Chernacoff interjects, "even a libertarian might allow for some circumstances where it's justifiable to limit a person's liberty. A well-known principle, the harm principle, says: Interference with an individual's freedom or liberty of action can be justified when there's a strong likelihood of harm to others."

"Here we go with the philosophy again," one nurse whispers to another.

Teddi ignores the whispering and continues: "The harm principle could justify temporarily detaining a person who poses a likely threat to others. It could not justify detaining someone believed to be a danger only to himself, however."

"What about the threat to others from having AIDS? Isn't that as much a threat of harm as wielding a gun or a knife?" a committee member asks.

"It's worse! Dying of AIDS is horrible! One bullet to the brain and you're dead, but with AIDS you linger on and on and on, waste away, get pneumonia, go blind, and become demented."

"The comparison is all wrong. If you're shot in the chest or the head, there's a high likelihood you'll die. If you have one or even a few sexual encounters with an HIV-infected person, there's a minuscule probability of becoming infected."

"Does anyone really know these statistics? Or are you just making it all up? I always thought, one contact and you've had it!"

"Order, order!" Ira Becker calls out. He turns to an infectious disease specialist on the committee. "Dick, what about these numbers?"

"It's complicated. There's a greater chance that a man will transmit AIDS to a woman than that a woman will infect a man. But even that depends. If a man has venereal disease or open sores in the genital area, he may have a 5 to 10 percent chance of acquiring the infection from only one act of intercourse with an infected woman. If he's free of venereal disease, the chance of infection is only a small fraction of 1 percent. The rate of infection in women is extremely variable. Cases have been reported in which a single sexual act with an infected man is believed to have transmitted the virus to a woman; other women have had unprotected sex with an infected partner for years without acquiring the infection herself. There are reliable data showing that anal intercourse in both sexes has a greater probability of transmitting the virus. One piece of research is looking for cofactors, circumstances that could explain why some people are susceptible to being infected by only a limited exposure, while other people seem highly resistant. That's about as precise as we can get at this time."

"Where does that leave us?" a social worker asks. "With such a wide variation, who can say if the likelihood of spreading the AIDS virus is high enough for us to detain an infected person?"

"It's not the simple fact of a person's being infected that counts here," the infectious disease specialist says. "It's *behavior* that spreads the AIDS virus, and only certain kinds of behavior. In order to justify isolating someone known to be HIV-positive, we have to know a lot more about the individual. Does he or she share needles? How likely or unlikely is it that the patient will change his or her life-style? Or enter a drug treatment program? Is the person unwilling to use condoms, now that HIV infection has been diagnosed? We would have to know these things, at least, even to begin to think of isolating an HIV-infected person. Does anyone here suggest we go down the road taken in Cuba?"

"What road is that?"

"They're quarantining everyone who's HIV-positive, putting them all in a special colony."

"Not quarantining, *isolating*. Quarantine is for a specific, limited period of time. Isolation can be for life."

"I hear the facilities aren't bad, though. Nicer than some of the hovels poor Cubans live in."

"I don't think anyone here is suggesting we isolate all HIV-positive people," Dr. Becker says. "We're discussing a certain kind of individual, like the patient on 9 South who's been having sex with other patients. If she does that inside the hospital, it's obvious she's going to do it when she gets out."

"Dr. Diaz, is there any consensus among psychiatrists on this question? What does the literature say?"

"I think psychiatrists in general are as confused and ambivalent as other people. I did come across one article, though, when I was preparing for this meeting. The author discusses civil commitment of mentally ill patients with HIV infection. Wait, I have a xeroxed copy here—yes, here's what it says:

> Civil commitment may be an appropriate response to the mentally ill patient who poses a danger to others by engaging in behaviors with a high risk of HIV transmission. . . . just as an acutely psychotic patient who expressed homicidal ideation and possessed a weapon would be involuntarily committed, so might a psychotic patient known to be HIV-positive who expressed a desire to spread the disease to others via sexual contact or shared needles. The physician must clearly understand, however, that the basis for commitment is not the patient's HIV status or sexual behavior, but the patient's mental illness that creates danger to others."[8]

"Teddi, can you enlighten us about any of this? What do ethicists have to say about this sort of dilemma?"

"The ethical principle is clear, but the problem lies in applying it," the bioethicist suggests. "A danger to the public health generally, or to specific individuals, justifies taking the appropriate steps—either involuntary commitment or detaining a patient already in the hospital. It's easier to state this ethical conclusion than it is to specify the particular circumstances in which detention or involuntary commitment would be justified. To make a sound decision, clinicians need to have general expertise in the relevant mental health field; they need to be skilled in making clinical judgments in particular cases; and they should have ethical sensitivity and commitment to the rights of mental patients. Isolation or detention of HIV-positive individuals who are obviously unwilling or clearly unable to refrain from continuing a pattern of unprotected sexual relations can be ethically justified, according to the harm principle. But where there is no reliable means of predicting or identifying such people, the harm principle can't be readily applied."

"As usual, an ethical principle tells us what to do in general, but not in particular," one physician complains.

"But we have arrived at a plan for this patient," says Joshua Gold. "I've already said what we'd do about discharge or transfer to a psychiatric hospital. While she's still here, I don't think we can isolate her, but we can place her under supervision. We do that with suicidal patients, so why can't we do it with a patient who poses a threat to others?"

"We have a staffing shortage, Josh, remember?"

A nursing supervisor speaks up. "I think we can arrange for a transfer or switching schedules of some of the nursing staff. I'll see that an extra nurse is provided on 9 South as long as this patient is on the floor."

"Thank you, Ms. Concepcion," Dr. Diaz says. "But let's not forget the other question we brought to the committee. Should we inform the two men who are negative that they've been exposed to HIV infection by a sex partner?"

Dr. Becker looks puzzled. "Surely, they'd guess who that person is. It would be impossible to maintain confidentiality."

"Yes, but isn't that what the law allows us to do in these circumstances?"

"The law refers to regular sex partners, doesn't it, Evan? These two other patients can't be considered regular sex partners of this woman. She had sex with them only once."

"Once that we know of," a physician observes.

"I've already described the law's vagueness. The wording of the law allows discretion on the part of a physician, but it also refers to a 'significant likelihood' that the sexual partner has been or will be infected. From everything we've heard today, the likelihood of that does not appear to be significant."

"I haven't spoken for a while," the hospital administrator says. "You know my position, that we have to protect the hospital. I'm appalled to learn here today that patients on the psychiatric wards of this hospital are engaging in sexual intercourse right under the nose of the nurses. If this ever leaks out to the media, I can just see the headlines: 'Patient at Mercy Hospital Seduces Schizophrenic Patients'; 'Patient Spreads AIDS by Having Sex on Psychiatric Ward'! One of these patients is only eighteen, and so impaired that his parents have been appointed his guardians. What if they find out about this? They'll sue the hospital for sure!"

"Another thing," a social worker adds, "the hospital has an obligation to provide a safe environment for patients and might be sued for failing to do that."

"Anyone can be sued at any time for any reason," Evan, the lawyer, points out. "And bear in mind that a hospital can be sued for violating the rights of a patient, as well as for allowing harm to occur."

"With all due respect," Teddi says, "this is an ethics committee. The hospital has an administrative staff looking out for the hospital's interests. It has a risk-management department whose function is to minimize liability for the hospital. And it has a public relations department looking out for the hospital's image. Our proper role is to protect the rights and promote the interests of patients in the hospital. That's what we should be focusing on."

"Well, that's just the problem, isn't it?" Ira Becker asks. "Aren't we trying to decide which rights of which patients should be protected, and whose interests count the most?"

"I agree," Teddi replies. "We've actually gone a long way toward doing that. I was only saying that the hospital's concerns about liability and its image are not the proper business of this ethics committee. Besides, if the hospital does the right thing ethically, it will probably lessen the chance of incurring liability or damaging its image."

Dr. Diaz asks, "Have we agreed that there's no obligation to inform these men that they've had sexual contact with an HIV-infected person? If we start one-on-one supervision immediately, there will be little chance of a repetition of what's happened, and from what we know about HIV transmission, the likelihood that the virus has been transmitted to them is extremely low. My colleagues and I on the psychiatry service will devise a plan for counseling the infected patient specifically in regard to AIDS, and we'll try again to get her to join the group therapy sessions."

"Sounds good to me," one physician says.

"Me too," a social worker adds.

"I don't know," a nurse says tentatively. "What if AIDS *was* transmitted during these sex acts? It's a fatal disease. People have a right to know if they've been infected."

"Telling them they've been exposed doesn't tell them that they're infected. They'd have to be retested in six weeks or so. And maybe again later on. All you'd accomplish by telling them they've been exposed is to scare the pants off them."

"So to speak."

"Still, they have a right to know they've been exposed," the nurse insists. "Only if they knew that could they make a decision whether or not to get tested."

Another physician speaks up. "There's another consideration. It's true, AIDS is a fatal disease. But there are some treatments available now to prevent opportunistic infections and to prolong the period before symptoms set in. People who know they're infected can have their T-cells monitored, and when the count drops to the point where their immune system is compromised, they're eligible to receive the current treatment, the drug AZT. Individuals who've been exposed to the virus but are never tested couldn't possibly benefit from this early intervention. As physicians, I think we have an obligation to patients to enable them to promote their own health whenever possible. This means we have an obligation to disclose to these men that they've been exposed."

"I disagree," another physician responds. "We took an oath to 'do no harm.' Surely we harm a patient by making him worry unnecessarily. If there were a way to prevent the infection from taking hold, that would be one thing. But as things stand with this disease, I think you do more harm than good by telling someone who has a very small chance of being infected that he's been exposed to the AIDS virus. We shouldn't dump bad news on patients, and worry them sick, without good reason."

"Isn't being able to provide early therapeutic intervention good reason?"

"Not good enough, in my opinion."

"Look, AIDS is different from other diseases," another physician says. "There may be a risk to *us* from patients who are HIV-positive. That's another reason for telling patients who've been exposed. They'll consent to be tested so they can know, and we can find out at the same time and be able to protect ourselves."

"You should be protecting yourself anyway," the infectious disease specialist admonishes his colleague. "If you use protective equipment only for patients you *know* to be HIV-positive, you're placing yourself at greater risk. What about people who have no reason to think they're infected but are HIV-positive anyway? And how about those who have been exposed but haven't yet seroconverted? They can infect others, but their blood won't test positive until they begin to make antibodies. We've been debating these issues since the blood test for AIDS was first instituted in 1985. The policy we adopted here three years ago is still sound. There's no danger to health professionals from casual contact with HIV-infected patients, but when a procedure involves blood or other body fluids, then precautions should be taken."

"Is there anything about the case we've been discussing today that suggests the need for a hospital policy?" Dr. Becker asks the group.

No one responds affirmatively.

"Okay, then let me review once more the committee's recommendations to Dr. Diaz and her staff. We concur in your plan to continue to evaluate Ms. A. for possible discharge, since there's no need for her immediate release from the hospital. It's agreed that additional supervision will be provided by nursing to prevent future sexual encounters between this patient and others on the ward. And I think the majority of committee members feel that disclosure to the men that they may have been exposed to the AIDS virus is not ethically justifiable or legally required. Did I miss anything?"

"Only that we're going to provide AIDS counseling and more support for Ms. A.," Joshua Gold adds.

"Of course, that's part of your clinical management of the patient. Okay, we've run a little overtime today. Thanks everyone."

❀

The three psychiatrists take the elevator together. Exercising great restraint, they refrain from talking in public about the ethics committee meeting. When they get off at the ninth floor, Joshua Gold glances into room 908 and sees Frannie standing inside, with her hand on Mustafa Moore's shoulder.

"Uh oh, just in time. Should one of us speak with her now?" Joshua asks.

"I will," Dr. Diaz replies. Gently, she escorts Frannie out of 908 and into her office. There the doctor confronts her with what they have learned about her sexual encounters with patients. Frannie is contrite.

"I know it's not allowed. I'm sorry. But I was really angry about your keeping me here in the hospital. I guess I got a little wild, having sex with these different guys. I'm sorry I broke the rules here, but no one was harmed. I use condoms now, you know. Ever since I had a bout of gonorrhea last year. Luckily, I wasn't too sick, but I got worried about STDs, started carrying condoms with me all the time. But it was too late for me with the AIDS thing." She begins to cry. "If only I'd been careful back then. It was three years ago. How could I have known then?"

Dr. Diaz comforts Frannie. The psychiatrist feels sympathy for her patient and relief at the news. She makes a mental note to notify Dr. Becker so he can give the ethics committee an update at the next month's meeting.

Abusing and Refusing while Pregnant

Two days later, as the daily group therapy session ends, a psychiatric nurse is waiting for Frannie to emerge.

"Ms. Amiga, there was a phone call for you during the therapy session. Your brother, Larry Roberts. He asked if you could call him back. He's at work. Here's his number."

"I have the number, thanks." Frannie goes to the pay phone and calls. "Mr. Roberts, please." When Larry picks up, Frannie says, "Hello, Larry, it's Fran. I hope you called to say you're going to spring me from this place."

"I wish I could. No, I called about the thing you asked me about. I'm in the office, so I can't talk too loud. Listen, I found out about Vinnie Martino, but I don't know if this is going to be good news or bad news. He's dead. He died a few months ago. I was really shocked, you know? A young guy like that."

"Oh God! Larry, who did you talk to?"

"I managed to track down one of his brothers. Frank was nice, but I felt weird hearing this news."

"Did Frank say what Vinnie died from? Was it an accident?"

"Funny thing is, he wouldn't say anything about it. I asked, but I didn't want to be too nosy. Frank really clammed up. Maybe it was an overdose. Didn't Vinnie have a drug problem at one time?"

"He sure did! That was what happened between us; I thought you knew that. He went to a drug rehab place, and I thought he was getting his act together. Then one day I discovered his works. We had one big fight, and I walked out."

"Hmmm. So, I'm probably right. Must have been a drug overdose. Poor guy."

"Poor guy! It's his own stupid fault!"

"Frannie, take it easy. I understand your feelings. But you know how it is with addicts."

"Yeah, I know. They go around ruining other people's lives. Anyway, thanks for finding this out. I really appreciate it."

"No problem. Look, Fran, I got to get back to work. Call me at home tonight if you want to talk some more, okay?"

"Okay. Thanks again, Larry. Bye."

❀

Frannie leaves a message with the nurse that she wants to talk to Dr. Gold, and later that afternoon he comes to her room.

"Dr. Gold, I'm going to ask you again to discharge me. I found out something today from my brother. The guy who gave me AIDS is dead. I know you and the other doctors thought I might go out and try to harm him in some way. I mean, you were right, I really was furious and wanted to get revenge. But he's already dead. So that's that. Could you sign the papers so I can get out of this place?"

Caught off guard by the information and Frannie's request, Joshua Gold pauses. "Ms. Amiga, I'm sorry to hear about the death of your friend. I'll have to talk with—"

"Sorry! You should be glad! He stopped being my friend years ago. Now what about my discharge?"

"As I started to say, I'll just have to speak with Dr. Diaz and Ms. Williams, and I think we'll be able to arrange for your discharge very soon."

"Good. Can't be soon enough for me."

Dr. Gold meets with his colleagues first thing in the morning and informs them of this new development.

Dr. Diaz ponders a moment. "I think the only reason left for keeping her here is gone. When she came in, she was evaluated as being a danger to herself and others. Then she was no longer suicidal, but we felt uneasy about discharging her because of her continual threats regarding the man she thought infected her. Now that that problem is out of the way, I see no reason why she can't be released. How does she seem to you now, Josh?"

"Sober and rational," Dr. Gold replies.

"But wait. She's HIV-positive." Blanche Williams says. "Isn't she still a danger to others?"

"Ah, come on! We've been through all that, Blanche," Joshua Gold says impatiently. "You know we can't detain an HIV-infected person simply because of the infection."

"I'm sorry, but I still think a sexually active person with AIDS is a danger to others. We've seen her behavior right here in the hospital. Shouldn't we be worried that she'll go out and place others at risk?"

"I don't believe so," Dr. Diaz asserts. "I didn't get a chance to tell either of you yet, but Ms. Amiga uses condoms. That's what she told me when I met with her just after we returned from the ethics committee meeting and found her in 908 with Mr. Moore."

"Marta, what do you mean *she* uses condoms?" demands Josh Gold. "Men use condoms, not women. Women may carry them around, but it's men who have to put them on."

"Not always," Dr. Diaz replies. "You may be surprised to learn that some women are very skilled at putting condoms on men, even without their knowledge."

"Oh, come on! With all due respect, Marta, as a man I just don't believe that's possible."

Dr. Diaz smiles. "I'm not sure you have to be a man in order to have some expertise about these matters. Believe it or not, the information comes from prostitutes. Following a study a while back, it was reported at some workshops I attended that prostitutes seeking to protect themselves from STDs and AIDS had become quite skilled in the art of putting condoms on men without their knowledge—or consent, for that matter."

"Well, I'll be damned. You never know—"

"But do we know that Ms. Amiga is skilled in that art?" Blanche Williams asks.

"What I do know is that she's careful about protecting herself. She had a venereal infection a year or two ago, and from that time on, she said, she's used condoms whenever she has sex," Dr. Diaz replies.

"Maybe that'll change now that she has AIDS. After all, she has no big reason to protect herself from less serious conditions now that she has a fatal disease," Ms. Williams says insistently.

"Blanche, you're too cynical," Joshua Gold admonishes. "This woman has no clinical symptoms yet. She's quite intelligent and has every reason to protect herself from other infectious diseases now that she's immuno-compromised. We'll hook her up with good HIV counseling here in the hospital, and I'm confident she'll take all the right precautions both for herself and any sexual partners she may have. I'm going to fill out the discharge papers now. Okay, Marta?"

"Fine," Dr. Diaz agrees.

Dr. Gold does the necessary paperwork and informs Frannie. In twenty minutes she's on her way home.

❧

Two months elapse before Larry and Bonnie receive a call from the Fecundity Center, informing them that another surrogate is available. Gloria Gardner has served as a surrogate for the clinic once before with no problems. Nevertheless, the clinic requires a psychiatric and medical evaluation for each surrogacy arrangement. Once again, the clinic sets up a meeting between the contracting couple and the surrogate. The encounter is cordial and congenial. They decide to proceed. And once again, eggs are extracted from Bonnie; they are fertilized in the laboratory with Larry's sperm; and two embryos are implanted in Gloria's womb. A successful pregnancy is achieved. So far, so good. When the time comes for the amniocentesis, Larry and Bonnie are nervous, but when the results come back, everything appears normal. Bonnie and Larry are elated, and Gloria is already spending her $10,000.

Early in the eighth month of Gloria's pregnancy, Larry's work calls for him to travel to a neighboring state. He and a colleague, Ray, make the trip by car, and on their way back rather late in the evening, they decide to get a bite to eat on the way home. They are about to enter a roadside diner, an hour's drive from the town where they live, when Larry glances through the glass doors at a long bar situated in front of the restaurant portion of the diner. Seated at the bar, with a cigarette in one hand and a drink in the other, is Gloria Gardner. Larry stops short and goes pale.

"What's the matter?" asks Ray.

"See that woman in the red sweater sitting at the bar? That's Gloria, the surrogate mother. She's carrying our baby. She's not supposed to drink or smoke. The contract prohibits that!"

Larry can't decide whether to go up to the bar and confront Gloria, or call her on the phone to discuss the matter, or call his lawyer.

"What will you accomplish if you confront her here?" Ray asks.

"Well, for one thing, she'll see that I know what she's been doing. She won't be able to lie and say she wasn't smoking and drinking. I caught her in the act."

"Yes, but what's the next step?"

"I don't know. Maybe I should talk this over with Bonnie; she's always more logical about these things. Besides, she ought to know about this, too. We probably should think this through together."

"Sounds right to me. I guess you don't want this surrogate mother to see you now, right? Let's go someplace else for a hamburger."

❀

Larry arrives home around 11:30 that night and finds Bonnie awake, watching television.

"Hi, hon, how was your trip?"

"Okay, but wait'll you hear this. Ray and I stopped at the Belmont Diner on our way home, and who do you think was sitting at the bar? Gloria Gardner!"

"What a coincidence! Did you talk to her?"

"Bonnie, I don't think you get the point."

"What point? You saw her sitting at the bar."

"She was *drinking*. And smoking, too."

"Drinking alcohol, you mean?"

"Of course, drinking alcohol! What else do people drink at bars?"

"Some people drink Diet Coke. Me, for example."

"Well, Gloria Gardner had a martini in her hand. With a little pickled onion in it."

"Then it was a Gibson, not a martini."

"Bonnie, is your head on the moon? This woman is carrying our baby!"

"I know, Larry, I'm not happy about this either. But what should we do about it? What *can* we do about it? You say she was smoking, too?"

"Yeah, and for all we know maybe she goes home and smokes pot and snorts coke!"

"You don't have to blow this up; what she's doing already is bad enough."

"Right, and it violates the contract."

"Maybe we should hire a private detective."

"That's a possibility. But I really think we need to ask a lawyer. We all signed a contract, so it's a legal matter. I'd feel better if we got a lawyer's advice."

"I agree, but lawyers cost money," Bonnie says. "I'm more worried about our baby's health, but we can't ignore the added expense of a lawyer. They don't come cheap."

"Why don't we go back to Professor Blackstein? He was very helpful in telling us about the reproductive laws, and he didn't charge us a cent."

"Yes, but he wasn't really representing us, just giving us information. I'd feel more comfortable using Mr. Alexis. He drew up our wills and represented us when we bought this house. I trust him. And I don't think he charges an exhorbitant fee."

"That's fine with me. I'll call him first thing in the morning."

The next day Larry sets up an appointment to meet with Mr. Alexis in his office on Saturday morning. Larry and Bonnie bring the surrogacy agreement with them. Larry begins: "As I mentioned over the phone, we have this problem with a woman we hired as a surrogate mother. She's breaking our contract. We want to know what we can do about it."

"You brought a copy of the contract?"

"Yes, right here," Larry pulls out an envelope and removes the surrogacy agreement.

"Let's have a look." Mr. Alexis skims the contract and stops when he comes to clause 12. He begins to read aloud.

" 'Gloria Gardner, Surrogate, agrees to adhere to all medical instructions given to her by the physician performing the implantation and responsible for delivering medical care to her during pregnancy. Gloria Gardner also agrees not to smoke cigarettes, drink alcoholic beverages, use illegal drugs, or take nonprescription medications or prescribed medications without written consent from her physician.'[1] That's certainly clear enough. You say you actually saw her drinking alcohol and smoking a cigarette?"

"Yes, as I told you over the phone, she was sitting at a bar with a martini in one hand and a cigarette in the other."

"A Gibson," Bonnie corrects Larry.

Larry glares at her. Mr. Alexis looks puzzled but continues to question Larry. "Did you ascertain that the liquid in the glass was actually alcohol?"

"Of course not! I just assumed it; anyone would. People don't sit at bars drinking water with a pickled onion out of a martini glass."

"How about the cigarette? Did you actually see her puffing it?"

"Why yes, well—no, I guess not. What are you driving at?"

"I have to think about what will stand up under cross-examination. The woman could make the defense that she wasn't drinking alcohol, and that she was only holding the cigarette, not smoking it."

"Isn't that a little ridiculous?" Larry asks.

"Not entirely," Mr. Alexis replies. "When I stopped smoking I sometimes held an unlit cigarette and at other times a lighted cigarette. It was familiar having a cigarette in my hand, and it was part of the smoking cessation program."

"I didn't stick around long enough to check out all the details. Maybe I didn't look carefully enough, I don't know. I was upset."

"I can understand that," Mr. Alexis replies.

"Does one single act violate the whole contract?" Bonnie asks.

"I'm sorry, I don't get your question," Mr. Alexis says.

"I mean, the contract says the surrogate mustn't drink or smoke. What if she does it only once? What if this was the only time? Does it count as a violation?"

"Absolutely," Mr. Alexis replies.

"She could never prove it was the only time," Larry observes. "People don't smoke just one cigarette or have only one drink for a whole nine months."

"The burden of proof would be on us, however, to show that there were other times. You witnessed her smoking and drinking on only one occasion."

"Well, what can we do about this?" Larry inquires. "Does the contract say what's supposed to happen when the surrogate violates something in it?"

Mr. Alexis pauses. "Apparently not. This isn't really my specialty in legal practice, as you know. To tell the truth, I'm not sure if it's anyone's specialty. We're dealing with an entirely new area of law in these surrogacy contracts. But I can tell you, the penalty for breaching a contract isn't always included in the contract itself. If we treat this like any other service contract, the person who breaches the contract should be required to pay damages."

"What do you mean, *damages*?" Larry sputters. "It's a damaged baby I'm worried about! Maybe we should urge Gloria to have an abortion."

"Larry, what are you saying!" Bonnie exclaims. "Our baby is more than seven and a half months old—gestational age, I mean. It's illegal to have an abortion at that stage of pregnancy. What's more, it's immoral. Wrong, wrong, wrong!"

"I guess you're right about that," Larry admits, calming down. "But look, maybe no real harm has been done yet to the baby. Getting Gloria to pay money damages isn't the point. The point is to make sure we have a healthy baby. I want to be certain Gloria doesn't smoke another cigarette or take another drink during this pregnancy." He turns to the lawyer. "How can we do that?"

"Hmmm," Mr. Alexis muses. "I suppose you could hire a private detective to tail her."

"Hey, Bon, you could've been a lawyer!" Larry turns to Mr. Alexis. "My wife suggested the same thing when I came home and told her what I saw."

"Yes, and now I'm thinking about it again," Bonnie says. "I'm not sure what good it would do. If we hired a detective to spy on Gloria, it would only tell us whether or not she's smoking or drinking; it wouldn't stop her from doing it. Besides, what if she does it in her bedroom? Or her bathroom?"

Mr. Alexis brightens. "You know, I remember reading about a case in California last year. The woman was taking drugs and not following her doctor's orders, and they tried to put her in jail for the rest of her pregnancy. I don't remember the details, but maybe we have a precedent there."

"Have Gloria put in jail? Isn't that a little extreme?" Bonnie asks.

"It's our baby!" Larry retorts. "Don't you want her to be perfect?"

"I'll tell you what," Mr. Alexis suggests, "let me find out more about what sorts of cases have come to court and how they were decided. It's silly to sit here and speculate before doing the proper legal research. Give me a few days—a week, say—and I'll get back to you."

"A week!" Larry complains. "That's too long. By that time, our baby could have fetal alcohol syndrome!"

"Not likely," Mr. Alexis replies. "It's the best I can do. Yours isn't the only case I'm working on, you know."

"I guess we can live with that," Bonnie says. "But if you *can* get to it any sooner, would you do it, please?"

"Of course. I'll give you a call as soon as I can." Mr. Alexis shakes hands with Bonnie and Larry and ushers them out.

As soon as he has a block of time to devote to the research, Mr. Alexis gathers as much literature as he can find about pregnant women and substance abuse. He learns that there is a growing movement, joined by physicians, prosecutors, legislators, and others, to incarcerate or to indict as criminals women who use drugs or abuse alcohol during pregnancy. This movement is not confined to the use of illegal substances; though alcohol and prescription drugs are legal, they can cause problems for an infant as bad as or even worse than various illegal substances.

Mr. Alexis finds the case he had tried to remember during his conversation with Larry and Bonnie. The pregnant woman is referred to in written reports as Pamela Rae Stewart and also as Pamela Stewart Monson. The 1989 case did not involve coercion before birth or, in legal jargon, "prebirth seizure," as Mr. Alexis had thought. Instead, it was a case of "postbirth sanctions," punishment after the fact—after the birth and death of the baby.

The twenty-seven-year-old California woman was the mother of two children and lived with her husband. Her physician warned her that she had a problem pregnancy and instructed her not to have sex with her husband and to seek medical attention at the first sign of bleeding. Mrs. Monson ignored both instructions and, in addition, took amphetamines. Following the onset of bleeding, she waited twelve hours before going to the hospital. Her baby was born with extreme brain damage and died six weeks later. The prosecutor brought criminal charges, claiming that her behavior violated a California law prohibiting a parent from willfully omitting "to furnish necessary clothing, food, shelter or medical attendance, or other remedial care for his or her child." [2]

Pamela Stewart Monson's prosecution was thrown out of court—but not on the grounds that a fetus is not a child within the meaning of the law; the California statute clearly stated that a "child conceived but not yet born is to be deemed an existing person insofar as this section is concerned." Rather, the ground for dismissal was that the law was not intended to apply to a mother's refusal to obey doctor's orders.

In reading further, Mr. Alexis discovers that the dismissal of the Monson case did not deter physicians and prosecutors elsewhere from seeking legal remedies against pregnant women who use drugs or alcohol. Also in 1989 another failed attempt occurred in Illinois, when a grand jury refused—citing "concern over the mother's right to privacy"—to indict a woman accused of causing the death of her newborn baby by using cocaine during pregnancy. In that case, after her two-day-old daughter died, Melanie Green was charged with involuntary manslaughter and delivery of a controlled substance to a minor. The case was brought by the Winnebago County state's attorney, who acknowledged after the grand jury's failure to indict that "the statutes we attempted to use are not the best possible mechanism for charging individuals involved in this type of behavior." He said he d now lobby the Illinois Legislature to make specific provisions in th w for this kind of prosecution."[3]

Mr. Ale n't surprised to discover that things went differently in another jurisdiction. A twenty-three-year-old woman in Florida was convicted in July 1989, also on the charge of delivering drugs to a minor. The Florida case was a nonjury trial in which the circuit judge made the ruling. The woman had given birth to two babies who had traces of cocaine in their systems. In 1991 that conviction was upheld by an appeals court.[4] The court's opinion stated: "Appellant voluntarily took cocaine into her body, knowing it would pass to her fetus and knowing (or should have known) that birth was imminent. She is deemed to know that an infant at birth is a person, and a minor, and that delivery of cocaine to the infant is illegal. We can reach no other conclusion logically."[5] On July 23, 1992, however, the Florida Supreme Court threw out the conviction; its unanimous ruling held that the state legislature never intended the drug trafficking law to be used against a woman for giving birth to a drug-exposed infant.[6]

Mr. Alexis reflects on this line of cases and concludes that they lack precedential value for the case he's working on. They all involved attempts to punish a woman after her child was born for using drugs while she was pregnant. He needs a precedent involving some form of intervention while a woman was still pregnant. He does come across a 1984 case in which a physician in Baltimore went to court in an effort to force a pregnant woman to stop taking drugs, but that woman was taking substantial amounts of Quaalude, Valium, cocaine, and morphine—all controlled substances.[7] Gloria Gardner, though in violation of a contractual obligation, was seen consuming only substances that are perfectly legal. Mr. Alexis ponders where to turn next.

"Honey, I'm home!" Gus Alexis calls out as he unlocks the door."
"How was your day?" asks his wife, Lou, who is also a lawyer.
"Frustrating. Remember the Robertses, that couple I represented a couple of years ago? Well, they've got some unusual situation now. It

seems they hired a woman to act as a surrogate mother, and Larry Roberts observed her in the act of violating their surrogacy agreement."

"What's she doing?" Lou asks. "Claiming custody rights?"

"No, thank God! Shades of Baby M! No, the surrogacy contract requires her to refrain from certain sorts of behavior during pregnancy, but she's smoking cigarettes and drinking alcohol, apparently."

"How did they expect to enforce the contract? Or to monitor her behavior during the entire pregnancy?"

"Beats me. But Larry saw her doing these things and came to me to see what could be done."

"Lock her up, of course. Incarcerate her. Order her to stay in the hospital for the rest of her pregnancy. Mandatory detox! Is that what you have in mind?"

"I'm researching it. So far, most of the cases I've found deal with trying to impose punishments on a woman who has abused drugs during pregnancy, and her baby is born damaged in some way. I haven't found any successful cases of prebirth seizure yet."

"Gus, you're the enemy! Here I am spending my professional life defending women from all sorts of coercion and abuse, and you're representing clients who are seeking to do just those things."

"Wait a minute, honey. I haven't gone that far."

"Yes, but isn't that what you'd try to do if you found some basis in the law? Otherwise, how could you defend your clients to the fullest? I hate to say it, but representing these people on this issue puts you on the side of oppression of women."

Gus Alexis groans. "Maybe I should've gotten your permission first, before agreeing to listen to the Robertses' tale of woe. I haven't agreed to take the case yet, just to do a bit of research and tell them about the state of the law in this area. Maybe you can help me."

"I'll help you by trying to thwart your efforts," Lou laughs. "But seriously, let me tell you what I know about attempts to coerce pregnant women. Probably the most frequent attempts occur around the time of birth, when women have been forced to have cesarean sections against their will. Women have refused C-sections on religious grounds, because of fear of being cut, and for other reasons—some rational, others irrational. But a C-section isn't the only medical procedure that doctors have tried—and often succeeded—in imposing. Pregnant women have been forced to take medication, such as penicillin, for the sake of fetal health. In 1982 a court ordered a pregnant diabetic woman to receive insulin treatment, despite her refusal on religious grounds.[8] Going back many years, Jehovah's

Witnesses have been compelled to receive unwanted blood transfusions, including transfusions performed long before the fetus was even viable; I recall a a case that occurred in Jamaica Hospital in New York in 1985, where a court ordered a Jehovah's Witness to be transfused when the fetus was only eighteen weeks in gestation.[9] 'Doctor's orders' during pregnancy have included putting on weight or limiting weight gain, eating particular foods, taking vitamins and other medications, not carrying heavy groceries, making and keeping doctor's appointments, and refraining from having sexual relations.[10] That's what's going on out there, Gus. I'd really hate to see you apply your legal talents to furthering this trend. More and more, and in new and different ways, women are being treated as fetal containers."

"To be honest, I wasn't aware of all these developments. I did know about the cesarean sections but not all these other things. In any event, this is a surrogacy case, and I'm wondering whether that's different from all the other cases because of the contract between the surrogate and the couple."

"Don't get me started on surrogacy, Gus. I think the whole enterprise should be outlawed."

"Well, maybe, but that's not what we're talking about here."

"It *is* what we're talking about. If surrogacy were outlawed, or at least, if these surrogacy contracts were held to be void and unenforceable, the couple in your case wouldn't have a leg to stand on."

"Yeah, I know. But right now there isn't any law in this state."

"A task force is working on it," Lou says. "One of the partners in my firm, Tod Nielsen, sits on the task force. I don't know how they're going to come out on any of these surrogacy issues, though. It's too early to tell."

"I guess I'll research the surrogacy cases tomorrow, to see if I can find out anything relevant to the Roberts situation. I have to get back to them by the end of the week."

"Good luck! Or should I be wishing you bad luck?" Lou responds.

❄

When Larry and Bonnie show up at the lawyer's office on Saturday morning, Gus Alexis begins:

"I'm afraid I don't have very good news. I did find some precedents for court-ordered intervention during pregnancy, but they all involved a pregnant woman bearing her own child, not a woman under contract to bear a child for someone else. Frankly, there's never been a case in which courts have intervened because of tobacco use or light or moderate alcohol consumption. I think the only point that may be applicable is the customary remedy for breach of contract. As we've already discussed, that would be money damages paid by the party who fails to fulfill her contractual obligations.[11] There is another possibility, but it's much less common: we could try to obtain a judicial order for what's known as 'specific performance' on the part of the person violating the contract. Instead of money damages, the usual remedy for breach of contract, the court orders the contract violator to do the specific thing that hasn't been performed. That's why it's called 'specific performance.' But as I said, it's a relatively rare legal phenomenon."

"Could we try it anyway?" Larry asks. "It wouldn't really be specific performance, would it? It would be more like specific *abstinence*."

"I don't advise it," Gus Alexis replies. "Think about it. Do you really want to begin an adversary proceeding with the surrogate mother who's carrying your baby? A contentious court battle could be worse for fetal health than an occasional drink or cigarette. And if you lose—which is likely—you'd have end up paying for the services of the surrogate's lawyer as well as for your own. It's not a wise maneuver, in my opinion."

"So what are our options?" Bonnie asks.

"You could ignore the matter and hope for the best. After all, many women smoke during pregancy, and it's only recently that doctors made the correlation between alcohol consumption during pregnancy and complications in the baby. It's still not established that occasional or even light drinking during pregnancy can cause any harm."

"I'm sorry, but it's not acceptable to us to just ignore the situation," Larry insists.

"Then the best option is to confront the surrogate with your knowledge of her behavior. That can be done in different ways. You could reason with her and implore her to desist. Or you could take a more aggressive stance and threaten her with a suit for damages if the baby is born with any defects that could be traced to her behavior during pregnancy," the lawyer says.

"We're back to damages again," Bonnie sighs. "We want to *prevent* harm from occurring; that's what we're really trying to do."

"Suppose we threaten her with these damages," Larry says. "How would we go about doing it?"

"You'd have to confront her with the fact that you saw her in the bar that night, of course. Since your aim is to get her to stop drinking and smoking, assuming she does it on a regular basis, you'd threaten to sue for damages if the child is born with defects. Those damages would be likely to be much higher if she persists in doing things that risk the health of the baby than if she stopped immediately. So you have some leverage with this threat, in trying to get her to stop."

"Mr. Alexis, how could we monitor Gloria's behavior to make sure she doesn't sneak a drink or a cigarette in private?" Bonnie asks.

"I admit that's a real problem," Gus Alexis replies.

"Couldn't we require that Gloria submit to a urine test or a breathalyzer test?" Larry asks. "After all, they're making athletes and all sorts of employees take such tests. Why can't we require it? Wait, I've got a better idea. Doesn't she have to give a urine sample when she goes to the obstetrician for her checkups? We could ask the doctor to have the urine tested, and that way we'd know what Gloria's been up to."

"Larry, I don't think it's wise to encourage police-state tactics," Gus Alexis advises. "Besides, it wouldn't be right for a medical professional to conduct such tests on a patient without the patient's knowledge and consent. An ethical doctor would never do it."

"Look," Bonnie urges, "why don't we just confront Gloria with what we've discovered, tell her we could take legal action because of the contract, and see what she says. I'd certainly like to avoid legal hassles, and I bet she would too. I agree with Mr. Alexis: getting Gloria upset might do as much harm to the baby as her taking an occasional drink or a cigarette."

"Well, all right," Larry agrees reluctantly. "What do you think, Mr. Alexis?"

"I agree with Bonnie. I think you should try that and see how Gloria responds. I'm available for consultation any time."

"Okay, thanks very much. Uh, when will you be sending us your bill?"

"Not until we've decided whether to take this any further."

"All right, then, we'll let you know what happens after we speak to Gloria."

On the way home in the car, Bonnie asks Larry, "Do you want to call Gloria, or should I?"

"You'd better call. You're more diplomatic than I am. And maybe a woman-to-woman conversation would be best."

"I agree, but I don't think I should confront her over the phone with what we know. Wouldn't it be better to do that face to face?"

"Sure, but you'll have to give her some reason for wanting to meet with her."

"Don't worry, I'll use a good reason. And I won't lie to her. For instance,

I could say we'd like to find out how she's feeling, whether she's comfortable in the last trimester of the pregnancy, and if there's anything we can do to help make sure that she and the baby are both healthy. How's that?"

"Fine, fine. I hope this won't be a big confrontation," Larry says.

The telephone conversation goes smoothly. Bonnie invites Gloria to come over for lunch on Saturday. At the appointed time, Gloria shows up at the Robertses carrying some fresh flowers. "I thought you'd like these, in honor of the new life we're bringing into the world."

Bonnie is touched. "Thanks so much, Gloria. It's very sweet of you." She puts the flowers in a vase and brings out some salads she has prepared for their lunch. As Gloria takes a second helping, Larry, impatient to get to their agenda, observes: "Eating for two, eh?" and forces a laugh.

"You do get hungry when you're pregnant," Gloria replies. "I'm starving all the time."

"How're you feeling?" Bonnie asks. "Besides being hungry, I mean."

"Good, for the most part. I get a little tired now and then, but basically, I feel fine."

"Have you been going to the doctor for regular checkups?" Larry asks bluntly.

"Yes, of course, why do you ask?" Gloria looks suspiciously at Larry.

"Look, I'll be straight with you, Gloria. There's no point beating around the bush. I happened to see you breaking the contract a couple of weeks ago. I saw you at the bar, at the Belmont Diner. That's why we asked you here, to talk about that."

"You saw me at the Belmont Diner? Why didn't you say hello? Have you been spying on me?"

"I wouldn't call it spying. I was on my way home from a business trip and stopped for a bite to eat. I could see you from outside and didn't bother to go in, so that's why I didn't say hello."

"It sounds like spying to me. You snuck up and watched me without my knowing it."

"It was an accident, I'm telling you. I just happened to go to that diner that night. It's not as if I followed you from your house. That would be spying."

Gloria becomes defensive. "I consider this an invasion of my privacy."

"Privacy!" Larry exclaims. "What privacy? You were in a public place. A restaurant. Isn't a person allowed to look at another person in a restaurant?"

"Of course, but when you know the person, it's normal to say hello."

"To tell the truth, Gloria, I was too shocked by what I saw. You were drinking alcohol and smoking a cigarette—that can harm the baby, you know that. The contract we signed says what you're not allowed to do and what you have to do while you're pregnant. I'm sure you're well aware of that."

"Yes, I am." Gloria appears contrite, and at the same time, defensive: "This is a free country," she adds without conviction.

"That's beside the point. You're under contract to us, remember? You're carrying our baby. That limits your freedom, whether you think so or not."

"I know what the contract says, and I've been living up to it except for this one time when you were spying on me."

"Come on, Gloria, we're not naive. People don't drink just once. They certainly don't smoke a cigarette just once."

"You're harassing me," Gloria protests. And then, more calmly, "I'm the real mother of this baby, anyway."

"What do you mean, the 'real' mother?" Bonnie enters the conversation. "This baby came from my egg and my husband's sperm. We're the biological parents."

"That's true, but it's not the whole story," Gloria replies. "I'm the gestational mother, and the gestational mother is the *real* mother."

Larry feels panic welling up inside as he recalls the Baby M case in New Jersey. What if Gloria decides she wants to keep the baby? He remembers reading newspaper accounts about all the surrogate mothers seeking to get their babies back. He also recalls the meeting he and Bonnie had with Professor Blackstein. Despite the absence of laws governing surrogacy, and uncertainty about how courts will decide such cases, Blackstein had cautioned that not all future cases are likely to be decided the same way as the Baby M case. For example, if a surrogate mother decided sometime during her pregnancy that she wanted to keep the baby, or made a pronouncement to that effect at the time of delivery, a decision might go in her favor.

"You're not the real mother the way Mary Beth Whitehead was the real mother of Baby M," Bonnie responds. "Mary Beth was artificially inseminated, so it was her egg that was fertilized by the natural father's sperm. It wasn't your egg that was fertilized by my husband's sperm, it was mine. That makes me the mother of this baby, just like my husband is the father."

Gloria smiles. "There can't be two fathers, but with this technology we've used, there can be two mothers. I've thought a lot about this with the baby inside me. I didn't know why you invited me here today, but I brought along some material I've been collecting. Here, read this." Gloria hands Bonnie a photocopy of an article with yellow highlighting. Larry peers over her shoulder as Bonnie reads the highlighted section aloud:

Once the embryo is transferred, the recipient contributes the gestational site and assumes the risks of pregnancy, and she should therefore have the final decision-making authority over the embryo. Because of her greater contribution and risk, and to provide certainty of identity and responsibility necessary to protect both mother and child, at the time of birth, the gestational mother (rather than the genetic mother) should be deemed the child's legal mother for all purposes.[12]

"But this is only what one doctor and one lawyer are writing in a medical journal," Bonnie says, her voice quavering. "Wouldn't the law see the biological parents as the real parents of the baby?"

"You're not the only biological mother, that's my whole point. I'm a biological mother, too. The baby's in my womb. I'm giving it what they call the 'intrauterine environment.' See here?" Gloria shows them another article. "Isn't that exactly why you're worried about my drinking and smoking? You're worried it could have a biological effect on the baby. That shows I'm a biological mother, too."

Bonnie looks distraught, and Larry's mind is racing. The conversation has taken a different turn from what they had planned. He doesn't know what to make of Gloria's little collection of clippings and photocopies and is afraid to find out more at this point. Confused by the shift in direction and not wanting to lose control, he decides that the best strategy is to calm down and treat Gloria as nicely as possible.

"Gloria, I apologize for accusing you the way I did. I guess from your point of view it did look like I was spying on you. But you know Bonnie and I care so much about this baby, we really want it to be healthy. So we were upset."

Bonnie chimes in, "Yes, and we don't mean to be legalistic about the whole thing. It's not the contract that matters to us; it's the baby."

Gloria softens. "I want the baby to be healthy, too, and I want to apologize for being so defensive. I've been going through a lot in the last few weeks. My brother got into some trouble, and I can't talk to my husband about it. I was in the bar waiting for my girlfriend to come back from the ladies' room. She's been giving me a lot of support. She also gave me the cigarette. I gave up smoking a couple of years ago, but she smokes, and just this one time I thought it would calm me down. Honest, this was the only time. And I didn't like the way it tasted, so there won't be another time."

"And the drink?" Larry asks tentatively.

Gloria pauses. "I've had a few beers during the pregnancy. I admit it.

But please believe me, I don't drink a lot, or often. If I drank three beers in any one week, that's probably the most I've had. I know I violated the contract, and that was wrong, but I honestly don't believe an occasional beer is going to hurt a baby. Just think of all the women who drank when they were pregnant before doctors discovered fetal alcohol syndrome."

"That's what our lawyer said," Larry acknowledges.

"Your lawyer?" Gloria asks. "You went to a lawyer about this?"

"We just went for some advice, that's all," Larry says quickly. "We didn't decide to take any action. You understand our position, don't you? We don't want to take any chances at all with a birth defect."

"I do understand. And I'm prepared to make you a promise. I won't have any more drinks, even a beer. There's only a couple of months to go, and like I said, I'm not a big drinker."

After Gloria apologizes, Bonnie and Larry are reasonably satisfied with her promise that she will refrain from drinking and smoking for the duration of the pregnancy. But with lingering doubts stemming from her little clipping file, Larry becomes even more solicitous.

"Gloria, I'm really sorry to hear about your brother. Is there anything we can do to help?"

"No, but thanks anyway for offering."

Bonnie finishes clearing away the dishes after their lunch.

"Anybody want coffee?"

"I'll have a cup," Larry answers.

"Coffee?" Gloria questions. "I read that pregnant women should stay away from caffeine. I haven't touched the stuff since the embryo was implanted."

❀

After Gloria leaves, Larry muses, "I guess that's the best we can hope for. She seems pretty open, and she left on friendly terms."

"Maybe we should call Mr. Alexis anyway."

"I was planning to, just to tell him how things turned out. Also, I'll mention those clippings she brought."

"Oh, the clippings. What do you suppose that was all about?"

"Beats me, but I hope it doesn't point to the worst-case scenario."

"Meaning?"

"Meaning she's getting it into her head that she might want to keep our baby."

"That's what I'm afraid of," Bonnie says.

"It really galls me, you know? Gloria was examined by that shrink at the clinic, what's-his-face—"

"Dr. Upton." Bonnie supplies the name.

"Yeah, that's the guy. What's he examining these surrogates for, anyway? If he missed the boat on this one, couldn't he also be wrong about whether she'll give up the baby after it's born? I know these guys aren't infallible, but still."

"Larry, all he does is screen the surrogates. I don't think the psychiatrist can make predictions about how the women will behave."

"Then why screen them? They told us at the clinic, they're very careful after the Baby M case. But a shrink should be able to psych out a surrogate, whether she's likely to break the contract, shouldn't he? On second thought, maybe not. That other surrogate, Patty Mae Smith—she didn't want to go through with the abortion at first, and the psychiatrist hadn't predicted anything about that."

"Psychiatry isn't about predicting, Larry, it's about evaluating and diagnosing. And treating mental illness."

"They're not so great at that, either. Remember when we were reading those news stories about the Baby M case? The experts disagreed about a diagnosis there. One psychiatric expert diagnosed Mary Beth Whitehead as having a mixed-personality disorder, and another expert—the guy who wrote the description in the psychiatrists' official handbook—contradicted the first expert's diagnosis. Anyway, I'm going to call Alexis, just to let him know."

❀

"Hello, Mr. Alexis, this is Larry Roberts."

"Oh hi, Larry, I'm glad you called. I just came across something of interest in yesterday's *Daily Law Journal*."

"I was calling to tell you about the meeting my wife and I had with the surrogate. Do you have a minute now?"

"Yes, good, give me an update on that."

"I think it's all going to work out. We had a few rough moments, but she apologized to us. She knew she was wrong. She admitted she's had a few beers—says she never was a big drinker, though—but she said it was the only time while she was pregnant that she's smoked a cigarette. I don't know if we can believe her on that one. Anyway, she promised she wouldn't smoke or drink for the rest of the pregnancy. She seemed sincere, and Bonnie and I felt we could trust her. What do you think?"

"Well, I don't know the woman personally, but your judgment sounds right. And as we discussed, it's better to avoid hassles and confrontations if at all possible."

"There was one other thing that disturbed us. Gloria, the surrogate, had a bunch of xeroxed articles and clippings. She showed us some paragraphs from two of them. It got us worried."

"What was her point, exactly? What were the clippings about?"

"She tried to tell us that she's the real mother of the baby. She called herself the 'gestational mother' and quoted from some article where they said the gestational mother is the real mother."

"Was the article about a legal case?"

"No, not that one. It was from a medical journal. One of the authors was a lawyer, though, and the other was a doctor."

"Larry, this brings me to the subject I wanted to talk to you about. I don't think it's necessary for us to meet again, but as your attorney, I feel responsible for informing you of any legal developments in this area. I'll tell you briefly about the article I saw yesterday, and I'll send you a photocopy. There's a case unfolding in California that seems to be the first one of its kind. A surrogate is filing suit to obtain custody of a baby she's carrying for another couple.[13] And it's the same type of surrogacy you're involved in, gestational surrogacy."

"Uh oh," Larry says, "I don't like the smell of this."

Gus Alexis continues. "The surrogate is claiming that the couple hasn't provided her with financial and emotional support, in accordance with their contractual agreement. Of course, that's nothing like your situation, so there's no analogy with the facts. But the important similarity is the gestational surrogacy. The lawyers for the couple are arguing that there's no genetic or biological connection between the surrogate and the mother—"

Larry interrupts. "Gloria insisted that she's a biological mother, too. She's giving the baby its 'intrauterine environment,' and that's biological, she said."

"That's part of what's in dispute in the California case, in fact. The surrogate's attorneys are seeking a declaratory judgment from the court that she is the biological mother of the child. However, there are a number of features of the case that make it quite different from your particular situation. For example, the surrogate is alleging that the contracting couple is guilty of 'fetal neglect.' They refused to give her a ride to the hospital on one occasion and didn't go with her on prenatal appointments."

"We haven't gone with Gloria on prenatal appointments!" Larry exclaims. "Do you suppose that makes us guilty of fetal neglect?"

"Larry, it's not clear that this couple is guilty of fetal neglect. I'm not even sure there is a defensible charge under that heading. I just wanted to let you know that this suit has been filed, and I'll certainly keep you abreast of developments."

"That's in California. Is the law the same in our state?"

"Right now, there's no law in California *or* our state that governs a case exactly like this. The suit there bases the surrogate's petition for custody on a section of the state's civil code, which provides that 'the natural mother . . . may be established by proof of her having given birth to the child.'"[14]

"Bonnie won't like this any more than I do! But thanks for keeping me posted," Larry sighs as he says goodbye.

When Larry relates to Bonnie the details of his conversation with Gus Alexis, they ponder whether they should offer to accompany Gloria on her remaining prenatal visits. Deciding it's too late to suggest that, and concerned that it could arouse her suspicions about their motives, they agree to do nothing further. They resign themselves to waiting as patiently as they can for the weeks to slip by until the baby is born.

Grappling with Patients' Rights

After she is discharged from the psychiatric floor of Mercy Hospital, Frannie Amiga resumes her regular activities. Normally rather energetic, she is surprised to find herself easily fatigued and lethargic. She telephones Dr. Joshua Gold, who told her she could call him at any time if she had any problems.

"Dr. Gold, this is Frances Amiga. You said to call you if I felt bad again. I'm calling because I'm tired all the time. It's two weeks already since I left the hospital, but I can hardly drag myself out of bed to go to work."

"Maybe your depression hasn't completely lifted," Dr. Gold says. "Feeling tired all the time is one of the signs of depression."

"Is there anything I can take to feel better?"

"I could prescribe some medication, but it might be better just to wait it out." Then Dr. Gold recalls Frannie's HIV infection. "On second thought, maybe you'd better make an appointment with a specialist. I'll refer you to someone in the ID group here at Mercy."

"ID? An identity specialist?"

"Sorry. Infectious diseases."

"You mean my lack of energy could be related to the HIV thing?"

"Could be. Let's let him determine whether your HIV infection has progressed."

"Does he have to know about that?"

"Of course, that's the reason for the referral. But don't worry. The doctors and nurses on the AIDS team are very careful about protecting the confidentiality of their patients. You can be sure they won't reveal your diagnosis to anyone except other health professionals here in the hospital."

"All right, then, I guess I'd better see the specialist."

Frannie makes an appointment with Dr. Richard Nordstrom, an internist specializing in infectious diseases. Dr. Nordstrom informs Frannie that he's going to test her blood to see whether her T-cells (lymphocytes that regulate the immune system) have fallen below the normal level—an indication that the immune system has begun to weaken and is unable to fight off opportunistic infections. HIV-infected patients are then eligible to receive the drug AZT, which can delay the onset of infections that are hazardous to people whose immune systems are compromised. Dr. Nordstrom performs a thorough physical examination on Frannie, orders the lab tests, and finds that her T-cell count has dropped below 400. He explains the meaning of the tests and prescribes AZT.

Dr. Nordstrom tells Frannie that the drug may not relieve her tiredness and also that it may have some unpleasant side effects. "But I suggest you take the recommended dose. If the side effects are too severe, we may lower the dose, or maybe try something else, but let's get started with this. Call me in two weeks, and we'll make a follow-up appointment to continue monitoring your T-cell count. Now, do you have an insurance form to leave with us?"

"Yes, I picked up this form at work. But Dr. Nordstrom, do you have to put in my diagnosis?"

"I'm afraid I do. I can't leave that section blank, and I can't lie."

"But I thought there was a law in this state that protects the confidentiality of information about AIDS."

"You're right, but only to a point. Disclosure to insurance companies for reimbursement purposes is permitted by the law."

"Sounds to me like the law is protecting money instead of patients."

"It's the only way we can get paid," Dr. Nordstrom says. "I do have to earn a living. But you don't need to be concerned; there's no danger that anyone you care about will be able to find out anything from the insurance company."

By the time Frannie visits Dr. Nordstrom again, her condition has worsened. In his discussions with her, as with his other AIDS patients, the physician feels torn between his two obligations as a healer: being truthful in providing complete information about his patients' current condition and prognosis, yet helping his patients maintain hope. This physician is flexible in his approach, individualizing his treatment of patients according to his perception of whether they want to be in full charge of their own care or would rather let him make the decisions. Dr. Nordstrom is uncertain about Frannie.

"Ms. Amiga, I have to tell you that your T-cell count is lower this week. Although you haven't developed any clinical symptoms yet, that's not particularly good news. Would you like to know more about your prospects at this point?"

"No. If there's nothing I can do about it, I don't want to know."

The next week, however, Frannie develops pneumocystis carinii pneumonia and is admitted to the hospital. She begs the AIDS team caring for her not to tell her brother and sister-in-law her diagnosis, but she gives Dr. Nordstrom permission to call her brother and let him know she's an inpatient at Mercy Hospital.

❈

"Bonnie, Fran's in the hospital again," Larry says to his wife.

"Oh, no! Same problem as before? I thought she was back to normal."

"I'm not sure what the problem is now. Last time she was on the psychiatric floor, but now she's in the regular part of the hospital."

"Hmmm. Did she say what's wrong?"

"I didn't talk to her. Her doctor called."

"What did he say?"

"Not much."

"Poor Frannie. I guess we should visit her."

"Maybe we should wait a few days."

"What a terrible time for this to happen! I'm so anxious about the baby I don't have time to worry about Frannie."

"Yeah, I know. Anyway, the doctor said he'd call in a few days to tell us if she's getting any better. He said she's in the intensive care unit."

"That sounds pretty serious. People go into intensive care when they need to be hooked up to wires and tubes and respirators. Is that what's happening to Frannie?"

"Bonnie, I said he didn't tell me anything. Do you want to call him?"

❀

The phone rings at 1:00 A.M. Larry picks up the receiver and mumbles a hello. He recognizes Gloria Gardner's voice.

"Larry, I'm on my way to the hospital. I thought you and Bonnie should know. The pains are ten minutes apart, and I already called a cab."

"We'll meet you there, Gloria," Larry replies, instantly awake. "Be calm," he shouts excitedly.

Larry and Bonnie dress quickly and rush to the hospital. Gloria is already in the labor room when they arrive.

"Bonnie, do you think they'll let us into the delivery room?"

"Gee, I don't know. We never talked about that with Gloria."

"We are the parents, after all. Fathers are usually present, aren't they? I'm the father, so I have a right to be there when the baby is born, and so do you, of course, as the mother."

"I don't know, this is different."

"We should have put this into the surrogacy agreement."

"What about Gloria's privacy? We may have rights, but so does she."

The obstetrician emerges from the labor room and greets the couple hurriedly. "Mr. and Mrs. Roberts, we've encountered something unexpected. There's no cause for alarm, but fetal monitoring shows that the baby's turned around into a breech position. I think we'll have to section her."

"What?" Larry asks.

"Do a cesarean section. We remove the baby surgically rather than by a normal vaginal delivery."

"Does that place the baby at greater risk?" Bonnie asks.

"No," the doctor answers, "on the contrary. The baby is better off being delivered by a C-section; that's the reason for doing it. But it places the mother at a greater risk."

"This is the mother," Larry points at Bonnie.

"Well, I meant the woman having the baby. She's usually the mother."

"Not in this case."

"If you'll excuse me," the doctor replies, "I have to go back. The nurses are getting ready to prep Ms. Gardner for the section."

"Dr. Corbin," a nurse interrupts, "may I speak with you a minute?"

Dr. Corbin strides to the doorway where the nurse is waiting. "She won't sign," the nurse says.

"What do you mean?"

"Ms. Gardner, the patient with the breech, she won't sign the consent for a section."

"Oh, no. Not another one of those," Dr. Corbin says within range of the Robertses.

Bonnie and Larry rush over to where the doctor and nurse are conferring.

"What's wrong?" Bonnie's voice quavers.

Dr. Corbin looks distraught, uncertain how much to tell the couple and how much they ought to be involved.

"We are the parents of this baby, and we insist you tell us what's going on!" Larry cries.

"Take it easy, Mr. Roberts. I'll be right back."

Dr. Corbin disappears into the labor room. A fetal monitor is in place, and Gloria is panting and breathing as she has been instructed to do. "Ms. Gardner, the nurse tells me you don't want to sign the consent form."

"I don't want surgery. I'm healthy, the baby's healthy, and I was told I could have natural childbirth. I was told a C-section would be necessary only if the baby was too big to come out normally, or if there was some complication." Gloria moans and breathes rapidly. Then she resumes, "I don't want an incision, and I was told I wouldn't have to have anesthesia."

"Ms. Gardner, I'm afraid I'll have to inform the Robertses about this. They're in the waiting room now, and I feel they must be told."

"That's okay with me. But nobody can force me to have surgery. I know my rights." Gloria groans and resumes her rapid breathing.

Dr. Corbin is silently praying for some miracle to resolve this situation. She approaches Bonnie and Larry. "Ms. Gardner does not appear to want the C-section. She won't sign the consent form."

"Oh my God!" Bonnie starts to weep.

"I'll sign for her," Larry says. "Or better yet, we'll both sign," he hands Bonnie his handkerchief. "We're the parents of the baby, and the baby needs to be protected, right? Besides, how can that woman be rational when she's in labor? We'll sign for her."

"I'm afraid that's not possible," Dr. Corbin says. "Only the patient herself can sign for a surgical procedure."

"Even when she's in labor? You mean to say doctors are powerless to do what it takes to save a baby when an irrational woman refuses a cesarean section? That's crazy!" Larry exclaims.

"Uh, some physicians in cases like this try to get a court order for a C-section," Dr. Corbin explains. "But I'm very reluctant to coerce this patient in that way," she adds.

"Aha! I knew there was something you could do. We want a court order." Larry looks at Bonnie for approval. Bonnie is shaking her head from side to side and sobbing. "Look here, if you won't try to get the court order, I'll talk to the hospital administrator."

"Mr. Roberts, it's the middle of the night," Dr. Corbin pleads.

"I know there's always a hospital administrator on duty," Larry says. "If anything happens to this baby, I'll sue you and the hospital and this surrogate mother up the kazoo!"

"I know you're upset, Mr. Roberts. We're running out of time here." Dr. Corbin looks around in desperation. The nurse beckons to her.

"Ms. Gardner is asking for something to relieve the pain. Do you want to order something?"

Larry takes Bonnie by the hand and walks over to where the doctor and nurse are conferring. "Did I hear you say she's asking for a pain killer? Give it to her! You can give her a shot to put her to sleep, and then you can go ahead and do the C-section."

"Mr. Roberts, please. You're interfering."

Dr. Corbin returns to the bed where Gloria is laboring. "Ms. Gardner, you want something for the pain?"

"Yes, please! I can't take any more!"

"All right," Dr. Corbin replies, and signals to the nurse. "Are you able to listen to me? Mr. Roberts is urging me to call a judge to order the surgical delivery if you continue to refuse."

"A judge?"

"Yes, we could try to get a court order to authorize the section. I don't like to do these things, but this is a very unusual circumstance. This couple is—are—the parents of the baby, and they will be raising the child. I think they have some rights in the matter."

"You're afraid they'll sue you, that's all," Gloria moans.

"I'm concerned about the baby, too. You're my patient, but so is this baby. The delivery will be easier for you and better for the baby if you will just consent to the procedure."

"All right, all right, I'll sign." Gloria gasps. "I don't want any more pain. Let's get this over with."

Dr. Corbin proceeds with the delivery after informing Bonnie and Larry that Gloria has agreed to the C-section. A healthy nine-pound boy is delivered. Bonnie and Larry are overjoyed, and when Gloria emerges from the anesthesia, she asks to hold the baby. She stares down at the red, wrinkled face. "Let me hold him for a while," she begs the nurse.

Larry and Bonnie are reluctant to leave the hospital, but they are exhausted and decide they'd better get some sleep. Gloria will have to stay in the hospital for an extra day or so to recuperate from the surgical delivery, but Bonnie and Larry can take the baby home in two days.

In the morning, after the shift changes, the nurses bring the babies to their mothers for feeding. The nurse asks Gloria, "Are you breast-feeding, Mrs. Gardner?"

"Yes, I am," Gloria answers after only a moment's hesitation.

The nurse assists Gloria in placing the baby at her breast. "There's no milk yet, of course, Mrs. Gardner. But the baby's sucking will help get the colostrum flowing."

Gloria experiences unexpected contentment as she nurses the baby. She is surprised at her own feelings.

When Bonnie learns that her son has been given to Gloria to breastfeed, she is jealous and angry.

"The nurses should never have given the baby to Gloria to nurse. I'm so angry we didn't leave instructions in the hospital. I guess we couldn't think of everything, Larry."

"It doesn't make a whole lot of difference, does it Bon? Tomorrow we'll be taking him home, and you can start him right off on formula."

"I guess I'm upset because she can nurse him and I can't," Bonnie says. "But you're right, tomorrow it won't matter anymore."

❀

The next morning Bonnie and Larry bring baby clothes and a blanket with them to the hospital. Larry has a camera around his neck, and their infant car seat is strapped in place in the back seat. Before picking up their son, they stop in to visit Gloria.

"It's that time," Larry announces with forced bravado.

"Gloria, how can I ever thank you?" Bonnie says.

"We'll have the rest of your fee in the mail this afternoon," Larry says.

Gloria looks hesitantly at the couple. "We have a wonderful son. I think

I've already bonded with him." Seeing a look of panic cross Bonnie's face, Gloria smiles wanly. "Don't worry, I'm not going to do anything. But I would like to visit him sometimes. Would that be all right?"

"We never discussed anything like that," Larry says.

"He can't have two mothers," Bonnie says.

"But he is partly mine. I did carry him for nine months," Gloria objects.

"I don't think we should discuss this right now," Larry says. "You have to get your strength back, and we have to take the baby home. We'll talk next week."

On the way to the nursery, Larry turns to Bonnie. "No way. I don't want any part of a visitation scheme. Robbie is our baby, and that's that."

"I agree. She has no right to the baby, or to visit him, or anything else. Next thing we know, she'll be asking to take him for weekends or summer vacations."

"Right. This isn't a divorce. She was our surrogate, and it's over now."

"Let's keep our fingers crossed that she'll forget this visitation thing once she gets back to normal.

❊

"Hey, Nick, look at this," Patty Mae Smith calls out to her husband. "Here's a birth announcement in the paper: 'Lawrence and Bonnie Roberts are proud to announce the birth of their son Robert, weighing nine pounds.' What do you know! I guess they must have found another surrogate. It doesn't say so in the paper, though."

"Of course not," Nick replies. "People don't want the whole world to know those things. They'll probably also want to keep it a secret from the kid."

"Do you think that's right? Keeping it a secret, I mean?"

"How should I know? I still can't get over losing out on the ten thousand bucks."

"And here I am, with my PMS worse than ever."

"Why don't you stop complaining and do something about it? It's months already!"

"I was planning to. But I still feel queasy about taking a lot of hormones. Besides, I heard the treatment is expensive."

"If it works, it'll be worth it."

Patty Mae makes an appointment with a doctor whose name was mentioned at the support group meeting she attended. The specialist employs an eclectic approach to PMS, prescribing a hormone treatment in conjunction with vitamin supplements, strict dietary restrictions, an exercise regimen, and daily meditation.

"I don't know if I can make all these changes in my life," Patty Mae confesses. "I never exercise. And it's going to be hard to stick to this diet with a husband and two kids around."

"Just do the best you can," the doctor says, reassuringly.

"No caffeine? Does that mean no Pepsi or Coke, either? How about Diet Sprite?"

"I'd stay away from artificial sweeteners as well as sugar," the doctor advises.

Patty Mae studies the long list of forbidden foods. "Oh, no ice cream! How come?"

"Well, it has refined sugar, which you should avoid. Also, the diet calls for no dairy products."

"There's hardly anything I can eat on this diet! No red meat, no dairy, no sugar, no artificial sweeteners, no caffeine. What's left?"

The doctor hands Patty Mae a brochure titled *Eating Right with PMS*. "Here, this may help you."

When the appointment is over, Patty Mae asks whether the doctor accepts reimbursement from the insurance company used by her employer. The doctor takes the form from Patty Mae. "I'll fill this out and the insurance company will pay my fee directly."

Patty Mae hesitates. "I don't want you to write the diagnosis on the form."

"I'm sorry, but I have no choice," the doctor says.

"Couldn't you put down something else instead of PMS? If my employer finds out, I'm sure he'll use it as an excuse to get rid of me. They're laying people off."

"There's no way they can find out. Insurance records are confidential," the doctor says.

"Maybe, but I don't trust them. Can't you just write down some diagnosis that doesn't sound like a chronic illness or a psychiatric problem?"

"I'll write 'periluteal phase dysphoric disorder.' I'm sorry, Mrs. Smith, but I can't lie on an insurance form."

Patty Mae faces a dilemma. She has to decide which is worse: risking that her PMS will be revealed, along with undergoing an elaborate and burdensome treatment that may not even be effective, or continuing to suffer the debilitating symptoms of the disorder. She takes out her checkbook.

"I'll pay you for this visit now," she tells the doctor. "I want to discuss this treatment with my husband."

That evening, when Patty Mae tells her husband what transpired at the doctor's office, he is livid.

"You paid her out of pocket? What are you, crazy or something? We barely make forty grand between the two of us, and you're going around writing checks to fancy specialists! I don't believe it!"

"Nick, what was I supposed to do?"

"Use the insurance form, what do you think it's for?"

"I don't want a psychiatric diagnosis on my records."

"You know what? You're paranoid!"

"Yes, in addition to having periluteal whatever-it-is."

"Look, this is getting nowhere."

"I have an idea, but I don't know what you'll think of it. How about if I go back to the Fecundity Center and put my name on the list of surrogates again? When I'm pregnant, the PMS is gone, and if all goes well we get the $10,000 we missed out on last time."

"Not a bad idea," Nick agrees. "It's fine with me."

❀

Patty Mae arrives at the Fecundity Center for her scheduled appointment with Mr. Epstein, the clinic's administrator. When she tells him her wish to try a surrogacy arrangement again, Epstein surprises her by saying:

"We no longer provide a surrogacy matching service here. Quite frankly, we're worried about liability, and also about our image. The bill in our state legislature that would prohibit commercial surrogacy is being debated now, and the outcome doesn't look promising. We're a respectable clinic, and although we don't see anything unethical in paid surrogacy arrangements, we certainly don't want to be breaking the law. If this bill passes, we'll have to stop making these arrangements anyway. We think it's better to halt the program now, so we don't disrupt any of our patients' plans or expectations."

"Could I be a surrogate on my own, though?" Patty Mae asks. "I mean, if I didn't go through the clinic, but say I advertised in the paper—would that be legal?"

"I'm not in a position to give you legal advice. You'd have to consult a lawyer," Mr. Epstein replies.

"Well, thanks anyway," Patty Mae says dejectedly. "I didn't think I was doing anything unethical when I chose to be a surrogate. I was just trying to help an infertile couple fulfill their heart's desire, and to make a little extra money at the same time."

"Well, there is one thing we could offer you here at the clinic. We're abandoning the surrogacy matching service, but we're continuing with all our other infertility services. Right now we're gearing up to expand our egg donation program. Perhaps you'd be interested in that. We do pay egg donors, but of course, not nearly as much as surrogates were receiving."

"What would I have to do?"

"Basically, it involves taking some hormones for several months to synchronize your cycle with the recipient's, and then having your eggs removed by a minor surgical procedure. It carries almost no risk. We're currently paying $1,000 to egg donors to go through the steps I've just described. One of the doctors here could tell you more about it, if you like."

"I would like to hear more about it. Could I do it more than one time?" Patty Mae asks, calculating how much she might be able to earn as an egg donor. "And what hormones would I have to take? Are they the same ones they use to treat PMS?"

"I suggest you make an appointment to see the doctor. I'm sure he'll be able to answer all your questions," Mr. Epstein replies.

Patty Mae makes another appointment at the reception desk before leaving the clinic. She can always cancel the appointment, she reasons, if Nick has a negative reaction to her enrolling in the Fecundity Center's egg donation program.

When Patty informs Nick about the program, he is puzzled at first.

"Is that going to help your PMS?"

"I don't know, it probably won't. I will be taking some hormones, but I doubt they're the same ones the doctor would prescribe for PMS. That's not the real point, anyway. It seems like an easy way of making extra money. Mr. Epstein said there's no risk, and who knows? Maybe these hormones will help the PMS."

Nick still looks quizzical. "Let me get this straight. You'll be selling your eggs to be used by a woman who's unable to produce her own eggs but who is able to carry a pregnancy. And the baby will be hers. That's just the opposite of what happened with that Roberts lady, right? Her eggs were okay, but she couldn't carry a pregnancy, and that's why she hired a surrogate. And the baby was hers. I don't get it. How can a baby belong to the woman whose egg it comes from in one case but belong to the woman who carries and gives birth to it in another?"

"That's the way the contract is set up, I guess. I don't know about that part. What are you worried about?"

"I'm not worried," Nick answers, "just curious, that's all. Will the woman who gets your eggs know who you are?"

"No. Mr. Epstein said the clinic keeps strict confidentiality of both the egg donor and the couple who receives the eggs. Here, I have a copy of the consent form."

CONSENT FORM FOR DONATING AN EGG

The Fecundity Center has instituted a program to provide donor eggs to women who cannot conceive. The eggs will be obtained from healthy women who volunteer to be donors. These eggs will be fertilized in a dish with the recipient's husband's sperm. The resulting embryo(s) will be placed in the recipient's womb. The program is conducted with the understanding that all parties concerned will respect the confidentiality of both the donors and the recipients.

I am in good health and have had healthy children.

I understand that I will be asked to take fertility drugs (clomiphene citrate or human menopausal gonadotropins) which may increase the number of eggs I produce. The major side effects are: bloating, lower abdominal pain; cysts may develop in my ovaries (these will disappear). In addition, I understand that after taking the fertility drugs I must abstain from having intercourse or use a reliable barrier method of contraception. There is a slight risk I may become pregnant and possibly bear more than one baby.

I understand that I will be tested, at no charge to me, for syphilis, hepatitis, and AIDS. I have been counseled regarding the significance of these tests. I will be informed of any positive test results and understand that they will not become a part of my permanent medical record.

The procedure for obtaining the eggs involves inserting a thin needle into the ovaries through the abdominal wall. The possible risks of this procedure are bleeding from the insertion site or from the ovaries. If complication deemed to be a result of the egg retrieval develops, Dr. ——— will provide care to me.

I agree never to attempt to discover the identity of the recipient or of a person(s) resulting from the fertilization of my eggs. I agree never to see or copy, either in person or through a representative, records concerning the recipient or any person resulting from the fertilization of my eggs.

If, by some means, I discover who the recipient of my egg was, I agree not to disclose to her or to anyone that I was the donor.

If I discover the identity of the person(s) who resulted from the fertilization and implantation of my eggs, I agree not to disclose to that person or to anyone that I was the donor.

I understand that I will receive a payment of $1,000 as reimbursement for my time and inconvenience.

I voluntarily and openly agree to donate my eggs under the conditions outlined above. I understand that the recipient and her husband have agreed to the same conditions of confidentiality.

Patient	Witness	Date
Physician		Date

"Well, it's fine with me if you're game. It sounds pretty scary, but you're the one that will have to go through it." Nick says after reading the consent form.

After some thought, Patty Mae Smith decides to enroll in the Fecundity Center's egg donation program as soon as she can get an appointment with the doctor.

❁

Despite the efforts of skilled physicians to combat the opportunistic infections associated with Frannie Amiga's HIV disease, her condition worsens. She develops AIDS encephalopathy, involvement of the brain that results in progressive dementia. After several weeks Frannie no longer has the mental capacity to participate in decisions surrounding her own treatment. She is on a regular floor for acutely ill patients at Mercy Hospital, with an intravenous line in her arm for the delivery of medications and nutrients. But she is not hooked up to a ventilator or any monitoring devices.

At a regular meeting of the AIDS team, Dr. Nordstrom poses a dilemma to the other team members. "We have to decide what to do about Ms. Amiga. She's been asking us all along not to reveal her diagnosis to her family. But now she's encephalopathic and can no longer give consent to treatment. She's stable at present, but it's apparent that she'll soon need ventilatory assistance and maybe other aggressive interventions if we're going to prolong her life. We can't do any invasive procedures without getting consent, but we can't just omit doing those things. In fact, I think we'd need consent to *withhold* treatments that would normally be given to patients with her condition. So what do we do?"

"Is there any chance she'll regain her ability to participate in decisions?" one physician asks.

"I doubt it," Dr. Nordstrom replies. "We asked for a neurology consult, and the assessment was that she's already too far gone. There's virtually no chance she'll regain decisional capacity."

"Well, if she's incompetent, the next of kin will have to be asked to consent. There's no other choice, is there?" a nurse asks.

"We could ask them to consent, but their consent wouldn't be informed if they didn't know her diagnosis. I'm wondering if this situation requires us to breach confidentiality. We have an obligation to our patient to try to administer appropriate medical treatment," Dr. Nordstrom says.

"Yes, but don't we also have an obligation to preserve confidentiality, especially when a patient has explicitly requested it?" a social worker asks.

A young physician speaks up. "Why don't we obtain consent from the AOD, the administration-on-duty? If we have no other solution, we can take the administrative route, can't we?"

"I don't know about that," Dr. Nordstrom replies. "I'm going to call for a consult from the ethics committee. We should be able to arrange it in the next day or so, before we're faced with an emergency decision for Ms. Amiga.

The following afternoon two members of the hospital ethics committee arrive for the consultation with the AIDS team. Dr. Nordstrom describes the case to them.

"The patient, F.A., is a thirty-two-year old white female. She has AIDS dementia but has not been legally determined to be incompetent, so she has no legally appointed guardian. Her next of kin are a brother and sister-in-law. Are they legally empowered to consent on her behalf? Here's our ethical dilemma. We need consent either to institute aggressive therapy or to withhold any medically indicated treatment. The patient lacks the capacity to consent. She has specifically asked that her next of kin not be told her diagnosis of AIDS. On the one hand, as physicians we're bound to preserve the patient's confidentiality. On the other hand, informed consent requires that the consenting party be properly informed about the patient's diagnosis and prognosis, and the risks and benefits of treatment. Giving that information entails breaching confidentiality. So, it seems, we would be violating an ethical requirement whichever way we act. One possibility might be to obtain administrative consent from the hospital's administrator-on-duty. What do you think?"

"Let me begin with the easy answer," responds Teddi Chernacoff, one of the two ethics consultants. "Administrative consent is not an option here. That's a mechanism designed for emergency situations, where a therapeutic intervention must be done before a patient's family can be reached. It's not a mechanism that can be used to resolve a case like the one we're discussing here."

"So we're back to the dilemma," Dr. Nordstrom says. "Whichever way we act, we'll be violating an ethical principle."

The two consultants ask for more details about the case, inquiring whether there's a chance that the patient's brother and sister have already guessed the diagnosis. Some members of the team believe they have; others are sure the relatives don't know; still others are uncertain. After a forty-five-minute discussion Teddi Chernacoff offers an ethical analysis and resolution.

"I think this case can be resolved without violating an ethical principle at all. As the ethical dilemma was presented to us, it seemed impossible to satisfy both the requirements of informed consent and the need to preserve patient confidentiality. In fact, however, the patient's brother and sister-in-law could properly be asked to give consent for a needed intervention without having to be told the precise diagnosis. They must be given the information *material* to making an informed decision; that usually includes the diagnosis, but it need not. The standard of disclosure in the law of informed consent has been interpreted by courts as less than a standard of 'full and frank disclosure.' It is the standard known as *materiality*— that which is necessary for a reasonable person to be able to make an informed choice. The elements that must be disclosed are the purpose of the intervention, what procedures will be done, the risks, the benefits, and any reasonable alternative therapies."

"That sounds like a cop-out to me," the young doctor on the AIDS team objects. "It makes a mockery of informed consent."

"Not really," Teddi replies. "I want to emphasize that in the process of obtaining informed consent, disclosure should normally include the diagnosis, but a case like this is a legitimate exception. The patient has stated expressly that she does not want her family to know. The relatives must be told, of course, that the patient is gravely ill, that in all likelihood she won't recover from this illness, but that her life might be prolonged by some measures. In answer to any pressing questions, you can truthfully reply that you can't disclose the diagnosis because the patient asked you not to, and you're bound by your obligation to respect her request."

"Then surely they'll guess what the diagnosis is. There's no other disease these days that patients want to maintain absolute secrecy about, is there?" the social worker asks.

"Perhaps not. But the point is, how can you maintain your obligation to your patient? You promised not to disclose the diagnosis of AIDS. You didn't promise to do everything in your power to prevent the family from guessing the diagnosis."

The physician consultant from the ethics committee makes an additional observation.

"There's another important lesson to be learned from this case. That's the value of holding a discussion with the patient herself while she still has decisional capacity. Then the patient's own wishes about future treatment can be ascertained, documented in the chart, and used to guide future medical decisions. In caring for patients with AIDS you often have the opportunity, at an early stage, to hold a discussion about the prognosis and what the patient would prefer. Because of the incidence of encephalopathy in AIDS patients, it can be predicted that many will lose the ability to be participants in their own health care decisions at some point in the disease. Some of them will no doubt express the wish to have their lives prolonged by aggressive treatments; others may choose care and comfort measures or transfer to a hospice."

"I agree, that's an excellent approach," Dr. Nordstrom says. "But it's so hard for us, as physicians, to talk about bad news with a patient. Even when patients know they have a fatal illness, we doctors have a difficult time discussing the dying process. Maybe it's our discomfort with confronting our own mortality."

"There are probably other reasons why doctors are reluctant to broach the subject of death with their patients," Teddi Chernacoff says. "But remember, this is all part of respecting the autonomy of patients. When there is reason to believe that a patient will suffer diminished autonomy at a later point in the disease, future ethical problems can be avoided by discussing the patient's wishes about cardiopulmonary resuscitation, placement on a respirator, or other life-prolonging measures. As this case shows, finding out at an early stage the patient's own wishes about current and future treatment serves everyone's interests and can prevent subsequent ethical dilemmas about how aggressively to treat, or about the role the family should play in treatment decisions. Family members may not override the wishes of a patient who has decisional capacity. And by the same ethical principles, a family may not demand a course of treatment for a patient who no longer has decisional capacity, if that treatment is contrary to what the patient himself or herself has requested. Holding discussions with patients about their future medical treatment is not only good ethical practice on the part of doctors; it can also make dilemmas like this one unnecessary."

The AIDS group thanks the ethics committee consultants for their advice, and its members resolve to initiate discussions with other patients before AIDS dementia sets in and renders them incapable of participating in health care decisions. The team asks the consultants if the ethics committee could help out by devising a living will for AIDS patients.

At the next monthly meeting of the ethics committee, Dr. Ira Becker, the chairperson, asks for reports of any consultations that have taken place since the last meeting. Teddi Chernacoff reports on the case of Frannie Amiga and the proposed resolution of the dilemma that involved obtaining informed consent from relatives without breaching confidentiality. The committee appears satisfied with that resolution. Chernacoff also mentions the AIDS team's request for a living will for AIDS patients, and Dr. Becker looks around for volunteers to work on that project. He then asks whether anyone has any new business for the committee.

"Yes, something came up on my service," Dr. Corbin, the obstetrician, volunteers. "We had a case two weeks ago of a woman who refused a cesarean section."

"That happens all the time, doesn't it?" one committee member asks.

"Yes, it does, but there was a special twist to this case. The woman in labor was a surrogate, having a baby for another couple. The baby was in breech position; the couple was in the waiting room; and the patient was refusing to sign the consent."

" 'Special twist' is the understatement of the year! Is this committee supposed to be solving all the most vexing problems confronting today's society?"

"Why, I think it would be interesting to tackle something new. I'm tired of the same old stuff."

"How quickly we become jaded!" Dr. Becker observes.

"Actually, I didn't mean to suggest that the committee tackle the special twist of surrogacy raised by the case. I'm wondering if we need a hospital policy to deal with refusals of recommended C-sections," Dr. Corbin says.

"What usually happens in these cases?"

"Well, it varies. Sometimes the woman is badgered and coaxed until she consents. Sometimes the labor goes on so long, she gets worn out and stops resisting. At other times we try to get a court order."

"What happens if a judge orders the section and the woman keeps refusing? Do you tie her down and forcibly sedate her, then do the section?"

"I wouldn't, but I have to admit that some of my colleagues would. I'd stop at requesting the court order. One of our younger doctors won't even go that far. He says a pregnant woman has the same right to refuse a surgical intervention as a nonpregnant woman."

"What's being done in other hospitals? Is the practice of forcing women to undergo surgical deliveries widespread?" someone asks.

"I brought an article that reviews some of the data," Dr. Corbin replies. "C-sections aren't the only recommended medical procedures that pregnant women refuse. This article reports a national survey of the scope and circumstances of court-ordered obstetrical procedures.[1] The authors found that court orders were obtained for C-sections in eleven states, for hospital detentions in two states, and for intrauterine transfusions in one state. Among twenty-one cases in which court orders were sought, the orders were obtained in 86 percent. Eighty-one percent of the women were black, Asian, or Hispanic; 44 percent were unmarried; 46 percent of the heads of fellowship programs in maternal-fetal medicine thought that women who refused medical advice should be detained; 47 percent supported court orders for procedures such as intrauterine transfusions."

"Under what judicial authority can a judge order these forced treatments?" the lawyer on the committee wonders.

"If you don't know the answer, Evan, how are we supposed to know?" Dr. Becker asks.

"He's a judge, isn't he?" the hospital administrator interjects. "Judges are supposed to decide disputed matters."

"My question was sort of technical," Evan says. "There are legal rules for judicial procedures, and that's what I was questioning."

"This article says that these particular judicial procedures are based on dubious legal grounds," Dr. Corbin says. "And the journal has an accompanying editorial by a leading authority on health law. Listen to what the editorial says: 'In the vast majority of cases, judges were called on an emergency basis and ordered interventions within hours. . . . The judge usually went to the hospital. . . . When a judge arrives at the hospital in response to an emergency call, he or she is acting much more like a layperson than a jurist. Without time to analyze the issues, without representation for the pregnant woman, without briefing or thoughtful reflection on the situation, in almost total ignorance of the relevant law, and in an unfamiliar setting faced by a relatively calm physician and a woman who can easily be labeled "hysterical," the judge will almost always order whatever the doctor advises.' "[2]

"Are you implying that these judges are wrong? The reason they order patients to do what the doctor advises is not because the doctor says so," a committee member objects. "It's because it's the right thing to do. Aren't these judges acting to preserve a life, in accordance with the state's interest in life?"

"Don't forget it's fetal life we're talking about here. There's no guaranteed legal protection for a fetus."

"There is for a post-viable fetus. If a woman isn't allowed to abort a post-viable fetus, why should she be able to refuse a medical procedure necessary to preserve the life of a post-viable fetus?"

"We're discussing a competent adult woman's right to refuse an invasive medical procedure. This has absolutely nothing to do with abortion."

"It may have nothing to do with abortion, but it does have to do with the need to protect a fetus from harm. An adult pregnant woman patient is different from a competent adult woman who's not pregnant."

"Sure they're different. One is pregnant and the other is not. But that's not relevant to the question of the right of both women to refuse invasive medical treatments."

"Could we have a little order here?" Dr. Becker pleads with the argumentative group. "I'm not sure where to take this discussion." He turns to Dr. Corbin. "Do you have anything to add to what's been said?"

"I would like to bring up another point in connection with this article. Someone here referred to 'competent adult women.' A letter to the editor accuses the authors of the article of 'skating over the issue of maternal competency.' The letter notes that 'maternal competency was established by a psychiatrist in only 3 of the 20 cases reported. . . . No evidence is given that the other 17 mothers were fully competent in deciding against medical intervention for their own welfare or that of their fetuses.' "[3]

"I would have thought we were beyond that kind of thinking by now. The person writing this letter simply assumes that refusals of treatment should automatically trigger a psychiatric evaluation of the patient. Although it's sometimes legitimate to raise such questions, it is a factual and moral mistake to construe as 'incompetent,' simply on the basis of their refusals, all patients who refuse doctors' recommendations," Teddi Chernacoff insists. "Not only that—the letter writer appears to presume that with more careful scrutiny, psychiatrists might well have found more—perhaps all—of these women less than 'fully competent' to decide. The attitude expressed in this letter is demeaning to women. It's old-fashioned medical paternalism in a new guise."

"It's interesting you should say that," Dr. Corbin responds. "The author of the letter is a physician from the United Kingdom. Paternalism in medicine is very much alive there, as it is in many countries outside the United States."

"You know, twenty years ago obstetricians would try to pacify women who refused a C-section, then just go ahead and sedate her through the IV without her consent. The change over these two decades marks a greater respect for patients' rights, as well as recognition of the legal requirements of gaining informed consent," one older physician observes.

"I'm sorry, but if there's a question of patients' rights in these cases, what about the rights of the fetus?" a nurse says. "It's the obligation of the obstetrical team to protect the 'vulnerable' patient, the fetus, which is incapable of decision-making on its own."

"I disagree," a physician said. "I would argue that there's no compelling reason to force competent women to receive medical or surgical treatment, whether or not they are pregnant."

"Not even when the woman is in labor and you have a full-term, healthy baby on its way out?"

"It's a fetus until it's born. Then it's a baby."

"You're trying to draw an ethical conclusion from a mere definition!"

"Once it's viable, a fetus acquires rights."

"Who says?"

"The Supreme Court of the United States, that's who!"

"Didn't we agree here that the dispute over forced cesarean sections should be kept separate and distinct from the abortion controversy?"

"Even if we're agreed on that point, it's still true that the fetus has greater moral standing later in gestation than in the earlier weeks or months."

"Order, order!" Dr. Becker pleads once more. "I see we're not going to resolve this issue here today. Should we appoint a subcommittee to draft a policy? Then we can resume the discussion with reference to a concrete document."

Teddi Chernacoff raises her hand. "I know that's the way the committee usually proceeds, but I'm very skeptical about whether we'll ever come to consensus on this issue. I certainly agree with the committee members who say that the question of forced cesarean sections should be distinguished from the abortion issue, but the two issues do have some things in common. One thing they have in common, in the words of the overused slogan, is 'a woman's right to control her own body.' That slogan has been used to defend the right of women to terminate a pregnancy, and in the context of forced cesarean sections it refers to the pregnant woman's right to refuse unwanted medical interventions.

"An equally important thing these two issues have in common is disagreement over the moral status of the fetus. So long as people disagree about when 'personhood' begins, or when a human life acquires rights—in particular, a right to life—there can be no agreement on the ethical permissibility of abortion or of coercing pregnant women for the sake of the fetus. I've seen enough disagreement in our discussion today to convince me that we'll never be able to agree on a hospital policy regarding forced cesarean sections."

"But we have to have some policy, don't we? We can't pretend there's no need for a policy when we have cases such as the one I brought to the committee," Dr. Corbin comments.

"I'm not certain about that," Teddi muses. "This differs from the abortion issue in our society, where it's necessary to have some public policy. Here, doctors can act as individual professionals, according to their best medical and ethical judgment. Of course, the hospital shouldn't sanction unethical conduct on the part of physicians toward their patients. But in situations in which there's strong disagreement, where reasonable, thoughtful people disagree, then perhaps it's better *not* to have a hospital policy that mandates or prohibits certain behavior."

"I don't see how that differs from the society's response to the abortion issue," one committee member argues. "Reasonable people disagree there, too, yet we have to have public policy."

"Yes, and from an ethical point of view, just where has it gotten us?" Chernacoff responds. "Public policy on abortion changes from one period of time to the next. There was public policy before the Supreme Court's decision in *Roe v. Wade*; there was public policy after that decision; then came the Supreme Court's ruling in the Webster case, and now it's shifting again. The U.S. Supreme Court is not deciding the ethics of abortion, that's for certain; ethical answers don't change from 1972 to 1973, and back again in the 1990s. Just because abortion was illegal before 1973 and became legal after that date doesn't mean it was ethically wrong before 1973 and ethically right afterward. Judicial rulings, just like political solutions, aren't necessarily ethical resolutions."

"That's a fine note to end on for today," Dr. Becker says. "But I'm going ahead anyway and appointing a subcommittee to work on a draft policy. In spite of your objections, would you be willing to work on the committee, Teddi?"

"Of course," Chernacoff replies. "As long as you'll allow me to say 'I told you so' when we reach an impasse."

"Should the policy deal with the special problem of a surrogate mother who refuses a cesarean section?" asks a committee member.

"I don't think that's necessary," Dr. Becker replies. "We'll never have another case like that here."

"How do you know? The sorts of cases that have come before the committee this year are different from ones we've routinely discussed."

"I'll leave it up to the subcommittee to decide, then," Dr. Becker says.

❋

"Larry, I thought life would be so simple and wonderful once we had a baby. I never imagined something like this would happen," Bonnie says as she shows her husband a letter from Gloria Gardner's lawyer.

"It says here she's going to court to try to obtain visiting rights and privileges. Well, thank God she's not suing for Robbie's custody."

"She couldn't win, could she? Remember what happened in that 'gestational surrogate' case in California a few months ago. I kept the newspaper clipping. The county superior court ruled that the couple who were the genetic parents—like us—were the only real parents. The judge gave custody of the baby to the couple. Not only that, the clipping says he rejected the possibility of three parents because it would be confusing to the child." [4]

"That's encouraging. But still, remember what the lawyers have been telling us. Just because a judge in one court or one state rules one way doesn't mean another judge somewhere else will decide the same way."

"I know you're right, but still, I can rest easier with that case in mind."

"Bonnie, we knew all along there was this risk. Let's not pretend we weren't aware of it. What are we supposed to do next?"

"Get in touch with our lawyer, I guess."

"On top of all this, we have my sister to worry about. I stopped by the hospital tonight on my way home from work. It's awful to see her just lying there with tubes and wires stuck into her, and a feeding tube through her nose into her stomach. The doctor asked me what I'd like them to do if she needs to go on a ventilator."

"What's that?"

"Like a respirator, you know, an artificial breathing machine. What they put people on to keep them alive when they're dying."

"What did you tell him?"

"I wasn't sure, but it didn't seem right not to put her on the machine if she needs it."

"Of course it wouldn't be right, if that's the only way of keeping her alive."

"Yeah, but she's not conscious. She doesn't recognize me, or any of the doctors or nurses. What kind of life is that?"

"Won't she get any better?"

"No."

"How do you know?"

"The doctor said so."

"How can he be sure?"

"He's the doctor."

"But if he doesn't know what's wrong with Frannie, how can he be so sure she won't get better?"

"He knows what's wrong but can't tell us."

"Why?"

"Because Frannie asked him not to tell us."

"Larry, is there something you're not telling me?"

"No. I'm telling you everything I know. When the doctor asked me about the ventilator, he also said he was under an obligation to Frannie not to tell us her diagnosis. He said she asked him not to, and it was his duty as her doctor to honor her request."

"So, it's going to remain a mystery."

"I think I know what she's got."

"What?"

"I think she has AIDS."

"AIDS! Frannie? Larry, you must be kidding. How could Frannie get AIDS? What makes you think that?"

"I kind of put it all together. First, she had that psychiatric problem just after the clinic told her she couldn't be a surrogate. She didn't tell us what they said, and they wouldn't tell us, remember? The clinic said it was 'patient confidentiality.' Right after that, she had the breakdown and ended up on the psych ward. While she was there, she called and asked me to find out about her old boyfriend, Vince. Remember? I get in touch with Frank, Vince's brother, and he tells me Vince is dead. Frank clams up and won't say anymore. Then Frannie gets sick and goes into the hospital. She told us she had pneumonia, right? That's one of the things people die from when they have AIDS. Vince used drugs, remember that? Drug addicts get AIDS. They pass it on to their sex partners. It all fits. Then, today, I go in and see her just lying there, all skinny and wasted. And I notice there's a red bag in the garbage can. While I'm waiting for the elevator, I see this notice posted about how to dispose of sharp objects, how to put all infectious materials in the special red bags, and a bunch of other stuff. Frannie is dying of AIDS, I'm sure of it."

"Oh Larry, how horrible! It's so hard to believe! Will she regain consciousness before she dies?"

"Not according to what the doctor said."

"Do you think the doctor would tell if you came out and asked him if Frannie has AIDS?"

"I did ask."

"So what did he say?"

"He just repeated that he promised his patient he wouldn't talk about her diagnosis to her family."

"Well, that's our answer. If she didn't have AIDS, the doctor would certainly have said no when you asked him, wouldn't he?"

"Bonnie, I really don't know. But I think you're probably right."

"Let's have some dinner. I don't feel much like eating, but we have to keep our strength up for little Robbie's sake."

"Yeah, and to gear up for our battle with Gloria Gardner."

❖

Two days later, Larry receives a call from the doctor who has been caring for Frannie. After another bout of pneumonia she was placed on a respirator, but despite the valiant efforts of the AIDS team she succumbed to overwhelming infections. The doctor advises Larry not to disclose the cause of death to the funeral parlor, since some undertakers have been known to refuse to handle the bodies of people who have died of AIDS.

Larry and Bonnie discuss whether to withhold the cause of death from Larry's parents.

"They'd never understand," Bonnie says.

"They just couldn't handle it," Larry agrees.

They decide not to mention AIDS. "We can say Frannie died of an infection the doctors couldn't cure. That part is true," Larry says.

"I don't know if it's really lying if we don't mention AIDS. It's just telling a partial truth, that's all. But what if they ask directly? Then what do we say?"

"Don't worry, Bonnie. It'll never enter my parents' heads. Who would ever think that a nice woman in her early thirties, not a druggie or a hooker, would die of AIDS?"

Devising Ethical Policies

The subcommittee charged with devising a living will for AIDS patients agrees that the document should present a full range of choices to patients. Unlike many standard living wills, which focus on the treatments a patient might wish to refuse, the living will for AIDS patients does not make the presumption that patients will want to forgo life-prolonging treatments. One committee member who has worked with AIDS patients observes that many of those who contracted the disease as a result of intravenous drug use are poor or indigent people who have generally lacked full access to the health care system. When they are approached with questions about what treatment they would or would not want, should they later lose the capacity to speak for themselves, many AIDS patients reply that they would like everything possible done for them.

At the next monthly meeting, a draft is presented to the full ethics committee for discussion.[1]

LIVING WILL

To my family, friends, loved ones, physicians and all those concerned with my care, I, _____, presently residing at _____ _____, and being capable of making decisions with respect to my health care, make this statement as a directive to be followed *if I become unable to make or communicate my decisions* regarding my medical care.

I am aware that I am presently infected with the Human Immunodeficiency Virus (HIV) and/or have been diagnosed as having Acquired Immunodeficiency Syndrome (AIDS). I have known about my condition since _____. During that time I have had the following intermittent illnesses:

[Please fill in the following space if relevant]:

_____

_____

_____

_____

I have been told that the infections and cancers associated with AIDS or HIV infection may be treatable, and that treatments are being developed for the virus itself. Still, I realize that my overall prognosis is poor.

Therefore, the following is my directive as to my future care:

[In 1–5, for each section choose the sentence (a) (b) or (c) that expresses your wishes; then check and initial it. In addition, read (d) in each section; if you decide to refuse food and fluids, check and initial (d).

The treatments you might want to refuse are:
   diagnostic procedures
   cardiopulmonary resuscitation
   intubation
   mechanical respiration
   antibiotics
   dialysis
   surgery
   blood transfusions
   other drugs not for comfort

If you want to refuse all of these treatments, you should check option (c) for each section.]

1. If I should contract an illness from which my doctors expect me to recover to my present state of health:

_____ [ ] (a) I want my doctors to prolong my life and use all medically accepted treatments or interventions, or

_____ [ ] (b) I want to refuse *only* the following treatments or interventions:

_____

_____

_____

_____ [ ] (c) I want no medical treatments or interventions except those designed solely for my comfort.

_____ [ ] (d) I expressly refuse food and fluids administered by any artificial means or technology.

The same four choices follow each of the conditional clauses in numbers 2 through 5.

2. If I should contract an illness from which my doctors do *not* expect me to survive:

_____ [ ] (a) I want my doctors to prolong my life and use all medically accepted treatments or interventions, or

_____ [ ] (b) I want to refuse *only* the following treatments or interventions:

_____

_____

_____

_____ [ ] (c) I want no medical treatments or interventions except those designed solely for my comfort.

_____ [ ] (d) I expressly refuse food and fluids administered by any artificial means or technology.

3. If I should contract an illness from which my doctors expect me to survive but likely at a significantly lesser level of well-being:

_____ [ ] (a) I want my doctors to prolong my life and use all medically accepted treatments or interventions, or

_____ [ ] (b) I want to refuse *only* the following treatments or interventions:

_____

_____

_____

_____ [ ] (c) I want no medical treatments or interventions except those designed solely for my comfort.

_____ [ ] (d) I expressly refuse food and fluids administered by any artificial means or technology.

4. If I am irreversibly demented and am unable to recognize or respond to family and friends:

_____ [ ] (a) I want my doctors to prolong my life and use all medically accepted treatments or interventions, or

_____ [ ] (b) I want to refuse *only* the following treatments or interventions:

_____

_____

_____

_____ [ ] (c) I want no medical treatments or interventions except those designed solely for my comfort.

_____ [ ] (d) I expressly refuse food and fluids administered by any artificial means or technology.

5. If I am irreversibly in a deep coma or persistent vegetative state:

_____ [ ] (a) I want my doctors to prolong my life and use all medically accepted treatments or interventions, or

_____ [ ] (b) I want to refuse *only* the following treatments or interventions:

_____

_____

_____

_____ [ ] (c) I want no medical treatments or interventions except those designed solely for my comfort.

_____ [ ] (d) I expressly refuse food and fluids administered by any artificial means or technology.

6. I would like to live out my last days in a hospice/palliative care program, at home if possible, and if not, in an environment guided by the principles of hospice care.

Yes_____ No_____

This statement is made after careful consideration. It is in accordance with my strong convictions and beliefs and based upon my legal right to consent or refuse care. I therefore expect my family, my friends, my loved ones, my doctors and all personnel concerned with my care to regard themselves as legally and morally bound to respect my directives.

I have read this directive, asked questions about it, and I understand it and have had an opportunity to make any and all changes in it that I might wish to make. It accurately reflects my intentions and wishes, and I am signing this document of my own free will. No one has pressured me to sign this document. I understand that I may cancel or change this LIVING WILL at any time. If I do not cancel or change it, this LIVING WILL/MEDICAL DIRECTIVE shall be effective for the duration of my life.

_____ _____
Date   Declarer Name

The foregoing, consisting of 5 pages, including this one, was signed and declared by the above named Declarer, in our presence and hearing, on this day of _____ , 19__ .

First Witness: _____
Address: _____
_____
Second Witness: _____
Address: _____
_____

Dr. Becker turns to the committee for comments.

"I think it's a fine document."

"I agree. I don't have any suggested changes."

"Me either."

"What if something comes up that's not mentioned in this living will? A new diagnostic procedure or treatment of some sort? Would this living will still be valid?"

"Also, who's going to present this living will at the hospital when patients can no longer speak for themselves?"

"There's another document to accompany the living will," a member of the drafting committee says. "This one allows people to appoint a health care agent or proxy to represent the patient's wishes at a later time." Copies of the second document are distributed to the committee.

DURABLE POWER OF ATTORNEY FOR HEALTH CARE DECISIONS

I, _____ , hereby appoint
Name of Principal

_____ _____
Name of Agent   Address and Telephone Number

as my Health Care Agent to communicate my decisions as known to that agent and as reflected in this document and to participate in all decisions about my care, to the extent permitted by law.

This health care proxy shall take effect in the event that I become unable to make or communicate my own health care decisions, as determined by the physician who has primary responsibility for my treatment.

I understand that I may cancel or change this designation at any time.

Date	Signature
	Address

First Witness: _____
Print Name: _____
Address: _____
Second Witness: _____
Print Name: _____
Address: _____

"We should have living wills available for all our patients, not only those with AIDS," a nurse suggests.

Dr. Becker asks the subcommittee members if they'd be willing to work on a general living will, and they nod affirmatively.

"I seem to be the only person who has a problem with this one," the hospital administrator says. "If we encourage patients to check off boxes on a form that says they can have any and all treatments they want, this hospital will go bankrupt."

"Bob, patients are being asked to choose whether or not they want all *appropriate* treatments, not any or all treatments. We wouldn't give a patient who's dying of AIDS a liver transplant."

"Still, I'm opposed to suggesting to patients in advance that they can have all of these expensive, high-tech therapies," the administrator objects. "Doesn't the hospital have any say in these matters?"

"As a matter of fact, the hospital is required to comply with the law," observes Evan, a lawyer on the committee. "You know, of course, that there's now a federal law—the Patient Self-determination Act, which went into effect in December 1991 and requires all health care facilities to inform competent adult patients of the possibility of executing advance directives. The law doesn't say anything about what specific form the advance directive must take; that's up to the laws of individual states. But we do have to tell patients that they have the right to make a living will or name a health care proxy."

"The living will is simply an extension of patient autonomy. By preparing a document, patients can express in advance what they themselves would want in the future, once they lose decisional capacity," Teddi Chernacoff explains.

"And I'm saying the hospital isn't in a position to give all patients anything they want," the administrator replies.

"Are you suggesting we start rationing medical care at the bedside?" a physician asks the administrator.

"If it's necessary, that may be what we'll have to do."

Dr. Becker intervenes. "This is a topic for a larger discussion. I suggest we stick to the details of the draft living will for this meeting. Once we have a document we're satisfied with, we can address administrative concerns."

With a dissenting vote cast by the hospital administrator, the ethics committee votes unanimously to approve the living will for AIDS patients. Dr. Becker says, "That was pretty quick. The next item on our agenda is another draft report from the committee that worked on the policy on forced cesarean sections. Did the subcommittee come up with something?"

"I hate to say it, but 'I told you so,'" Teddi Chernacoff states. "We couldn't reach agreement. Four of the five committee members were prepared to endorse statements from the American College of Obstetricians and Gynecologists' Committee Opinion on Patient Choice, which opposes forcing women to undergo C-sections or other medical treatment. The fifth member was unwilling to adopt the ACOG statement. May I read the relevant portions of that statement now?"

Dr. Becker nods, and Chernacoff begins.

"The Committee Opinion embodies three main conclusions. The first recognizes women's right to self-determination. It says: 'Every reasonable effort should be made to protect the fetus, but the pregnant woman's autonomy should be respected.' The second stipulates that the role of the obstetrician is that of 'an informed educator and counselor,' and states that 'the use of the courts to resolve these conflicts is almost never warranted.' The third conclusion quite clearly prohibits obstetricians from performing procedures that are unwanted by pregnant women: 'The use of judicial authority to implement treatment regimens in order to protect the fetus violates the pregnant woman's autonomy' and may lead to 'the criminalization of noncompliance with medical recommendations.'[2]

"Can we take a straw vote of the whole committee? How many would be prepared to accept the conclusions of the ACOG statement as a proposed policy for this hospital?" Dr. Becker asks for a show of hands. Eight committee members raise their hands.

"How many are opposed?" Three hands go up.

"Some people didn't vote," Dr. Becker notes. "How are we to interpret the abstentions?"

A physician raises his hand. "I abstained because I'm personally in favor of the ACOG position, but I don't think it should be hospital policy. It would coerce compliance from doctors whose conscience goes against the policy. That seems wrong to me."

Another physician volunteered: "I think it depends on the particulars of the case. Every case is unique. I don't think we can have a policy that treats all cases the same."

"But we need to have some policy, don't we?"

"Not necessarily."

"Here we go again. We had this discussion last time."

"Does anyone have a constructive alternative to propose at this point?" Dr. Becker asks.

A member of the drafting subcommittee suggests that the ethics committee's policy guidelines acknowledge the impossibility of reaching agreement on this topic.

"You mean we should issue a policy that says we have no policy?"

"Not exactly. Here's some wording we considered at one of our drafting sessions: 'A pregnant woman has the right to control her body. A dilemma arises out of a demand that she yield this right during pregnancy because some physicians cannot ignore the presence of a "second patient." Though it is morally questionable for a woman to refuse a relatively safe procedure that would jeopardize the fetus, it is also morally reprehensible to infringe upon the person, privacy, and/or firmly held conviction of an informed adult.' " [3]

"I don't like the reference to 'some physicians,' " a doctor objects. "It has the effect of demeaning those physicians who hold the view in question."

"Yes, but the idea of admitting the disagreement up front is a good one," someone else suggests.

As the committee continues debating the issue, Evan, the lawyer, is scribbling busily. Just before the meeting is scheduled to adjourn, he proposes the following statement for the committee's consideration:

Competent adult patients have the right to refuse medical treatment. This right extends to pregnant women. However, some members of society assert that the fetus has "interests" or "rights" that compete with the rights of the mother to control her own body. In general, the rights of the mother are clearly acknowledged to take precedence in early pregnancy. As gestation advances, it becomes increasingly difficult for some members of society to ignore the "interests of the fetus." Because of the dilemma that arises out of these opposing interests, physicians have an obligation to disclose from the outset if, under specified circumstances, they would be unable to honor a patient's wishes.

Because society and the law have not resolved the conflict between fetal and maternal interests, the policy cannot establish guidelines for action where a clinician's interpretation of the interests of the fetus are in conflict with the wishes of the mother. The clinician and patient, with ethical consultation, must seek to resolve such conflicts within the context of the doctor-patient relationship and resort to other means for conflict resolution, including hospital administration, when necessary. Every physician has the right and obligation to try to turn the care of such a patient over to another caregiver if the patient's wishes are incompatible with the physician's professional and ethical values. This course of action is ethically superior to the coercion of an unwilling patient.[4]

"That sounds really good," one committee member says.

"I'd have to see it written down before I could vote on it," someone else volunteers.

"Congratulations, Evan, I think you've solved our problem," another person says.

"Does anyone object to anything in the statement Evan just read?" Dr. Becker asks the group. Most shake their heads.

Teddi Chernacoff says, "I don't object to anything in the statement. But I do object to incorporating any such statement into our policy. The policy should endorse the ACOG statement and take a firm stance against the coercion of pregnant women. Period."

"I see we're not going to reach a consensus, so we'll have to put this to a vote," Dr. Becker says. "I'll have Evan's statement typed up and distributed, and we can take a formal vote at next month's meeting. Please submit any proposed changes in wording directly to Evan as soon as possible."

❀

Larry and Bonnie are resigned to gearing up for a court battle to prevent Gloria from seeking visitation rights with her gestational son. Their lawyer advises them not to initiate legal action aimed at being awarded sole custody of the baby.

"Why don't you lie low and wait awhile. With the passage of time,

Ms. Gardner will probably change her mind about wanting visitation rights," the lawyer says.

The couple finds it difficult just to do nothing. The lingering uncertainty creates more anxiety than they would feel if engaged in active opposition. Bonnie decides to contact Resolve, in the hope of getting in touch with other women who have used surrogates to bear their children. She learns the identity of several who are willing to speak with individuals who are encountering difficulties following a surrogacy arrangement. Two of these women have maintained ongoing relationships with the surrogates who bore their children. In one case, it was the surrogate who insisted on contact with the child, as in Bonnie and Larry's situation. In the other case, the rearing parents were so grateful that they offered the surrogate the opportunity to develop a relationship with the child. In both cases the surrogates have taken on a role akin to an "aunt" of the child. But in neither case do the rearing parents or the surrogate plan to disclose to the offspring the part the surrogate played in pregnancy and childbirth.

"It's like artificial insemination," one woman says. "That's normally kept a secret, and only under unusual circumstances does the secret leak out."

"It's like adoption," the other woman says. "There are many people these days who favor open adoption and telling all. I still think it's best for a child to bond with only one mother and father."

Bonnie is heartened to learn of the good relationships these women have with the surrogates who bore their children, but she is troubled about the secrecy aspect. What if the secret does leak out? Would that be worse for the child? What if Gloria insists on telling Robbie she gave birth to him, unlike those other surrogates who were willing to keep their role a secret from the child?

❧

One day, Bonnie is in the checkout line at the supermarket, rocking Robbie to sleep in his carriage. The woman in front of her is flipping through a magazine when Bonnie catches a glimpse of her face and recognizes Patty Mae Smith. They chat briefly. Patty Mae congratulates Bonnie, telling her she saw the birth announcement in the newspaper, and reveals her thoughts about serving as a surrogate again, along with information about the demise of the surrogacy matching service at the Fecundity Center. She also mentions that she's planning to become an egg donor at the clinic and wonders whether Bonnie would be willing to recount her experience of taking the hormones and undergoing the egg extraction procedure. "Sure," says Bonnie, "but would you mind answering a question for me first?"

"Not at all," Patty Mae replies.

"Your identity as an egg donor is kept secret, right? And you don't know the woman who receives your egg? So the baby never knows that the woman who gave birth to him isn't his real mother."

"She *is* his real mother. The child doesn't know that half of his genes didn't come from her, but that doesn't mean she isn't his real mother."

"Well, I'm more interested in the secrecy aspect. How do you feel about that?"

"As they explained to me at the clinic, it's just like artificial insemination. Men donate their sperm anonymously, and children never know. Legally, their mother's husband is their father, and that's the way it is now with egg donations."

"What if the child finds out?"

"How could that happen? I sign a consent form and so does the woman who receives my eggs. We both promise not to reveal our own identity and not to try to find out who the other person is. That's the way all parties want it. And it's in everyone's best interest."

When the two women part, Bonnie struggles to sort out the differences between sperm and egg donation and surrogacy arrangements. Her curiosity does not abate, and her quest for more information impels her to attend another session of the Task Force on Reproduction. The task force is debating several unresolved issues for its report on surrogacy and still holds monthly meetings. Larry stays home with Robbie while Bonnie goes to the meeting.

"We have three remaining issues to resolve before we can complete our report," Maura O'Brien announces. "The first is reaching a final consensus on noncommercial surrogacy arrangements. We've already agreed on specific recommendations prohibiting commercial surrogacy, but we haven't decided on what the legal position should be regarding contractual or informal arrangements where no broker is involved. The second issue is whether to treat gestational surrogacy any differently from the type in which the surrogate contributes her egg as well as her womb. And the third issue— the hardest, to be sure—is what public policy should say about disputed arrangements, when the surrogate wishes to keep the baby. Let's leave aside for today any other considerations, such as the features of a surrogacy contract—whether commercial or noncommercial—that require a surrogate to act or refrain from acting in certain ways throughout her pregnancy.

"We've distributed the minutes of past meetings and the staff report summarizing our conclusions on commercial surrogacy and our discussions so far on noncommercial surrogacy. It would be useful for us first to review the nature of the wrong involved in commercial surrogacy and the recommendations we've agreed on so far. Before formulating our recommendations on noncommercial surrogacy arrangements, let's take a few minutes to reread both sections of the draft report.

PROHIBITION OF COMMERCIAL SURROGACY
Staff Report and Discussion

There was much discussion and some disagreement among task force members over the nature of the wrong involved in commercial arrangements. Some argued that paying women to gestate a fetus for another couple was an act of exploitation. Yet it was difficult to identify the precise features that would constitute exploitation. Evidence gathered by staff and presented at task force meetings revealed that by and large, the women who have served as surrogates are not the poorest of the poor. For the most part, their personal or family income levels fall in the range of "lower middle class," rather than poverty. These data serve to rebut the contention that the nature of the wrong is *economic* exploitation.

If not economic, what sort of exploitation is involved? A feminist line of thought contends that simply the use of a woman's body as a "fetal container" can be considered exploitation of women. After considerable debate over whether that would warrant condemnation of surrogacy as a form of exploitation, a second ethical concept was introduced: degradation. The idea of selling oneself, or a part of oneself, or the services of one's body, might be construed as degradation even if not exploitation. The task force failed to attain agreement over whether a person has to *feel* degraded in order to *be* degraded. Some argued that people can be degraded even if they don't experience subjective feelings of degradation.

Agreement was reached on two fundamental points. "First, when surrogate parenting involves the payment of fees and a contractual obligation to relinquish the child at birth, it places children at risk and is not in their best interests. Second, the practice has the potential to undermine the dignity of women, children, and human reproduction."[5]

In the end, the agreement of the task force regarding prohibition of commercial surrogacy rested on the notion that the wrong involved is that of *commodification* of the procreative process. The task force listened to an oral presentation outlining the theory that there are some forms of exchange among human beings that should be prevented from being carried out for money. After considering analogies with baby-selling, selling oneself into slavery, and the selling of one's own organs for transplantation, the task force agreed that these forms of "commodification" are so morally unacceptable that they ought to be legally prohibited. The fact that our society is capitalistic and is dominated by commercial transactions of all sorts does not compel the conclusion that therefore, anything may be put up for sale.

The discussion that spanned three task force meetings resulted in an apparent agreement that it is not surrogacy itself that is morally unacceptable but rather its commercial aspect. Yet that agreement turned out to be only an *apparent* agreement among task force members. A split emerged in the group over the issue of whether all surrogacy arrangements are so undesirable that noncommercial as well as commercial surrogacy should be legally prohibited. Several task force members held that a policy recommendation should explicitly call upon the state to prohibit noncommercial as well as commercial surrogacy arrangements.

RECOMMENDATIONS

—All surrogacy contracts are contrary to public policy of this state, and should be void and unenforceable.

—Any commercial surrogacy arrangement or any contractual provisions in connection with commercial surrogacy arrangements should be illegal and unenforceable.

—Violations of this ban on commercial surrogacy should be subject to civil or criminal penalties, to be determined by the state legislature. The prohibition of commercial surrogacy arrangements is intended to apply to brokers or intermediaries, women who serve as surrogates, the contracting parents, and physicians or other professionals who knowingly participate in commercial surrogacy arrangements.

Pages rustled as the audience finished reading the first and went on to examine the second section of the report.

WHY NONCOMMERCIAL SURROGACY ARRANGEMENTS SHOULD BE UNENFORCEABLE BUT NOT PROHIBITED
Staff Report and Discussion
(For committee use only— DO NOT CITE OR QUOTE)
The task force came to unanimous agreement that public policy should discourage surrogate parenting.[6] There was, however, an initial difference of opinion among task force members about whether noncommercial surrogacy should also be prohibited or whether legislation should hold noncommercial surrogacy contracts to be unenforceable but not

illegal. Several members of the group argued that it is inconsistent to prohibit commercial surrogacy—even to the point of assigning criminal penalties—and yet to permit individuals who engage in noncommercial arrangements to go unpunished. In its discussions over a period of several months, the task force reached a general consensus that the commercial aspects of surrogacy are its most offensive feature and that those aspects should be prohibited by law.

To understand why noncommercial surrogacy arrangements should not be prohibited by law, the task force sought to determine whether noncommercial surrogacy should be viewed as morally neutral or, instead, as morally wrong yet not of such magnitude as to warrant legal prohibition.

Those who believed that the state should prohibit noncommercial as well as commercial surrogacy introduced several lines of argument. One is the notion that exploitation of one person by another can exist in noncommercial forms. What about the poor, mildly mentally retarded cousin who might be coerced into bearing a child for her relative? While recognizing that such instances of coercion could occur, the majority of task force members viewed this as an abuse of a family member that could and most likely would occur whether or not noncommercial surrogacy is made illegal. Not every form of abuse or coercion within or outside of families can be prevented or deterred by law.

A second line of argument holds that by permitting noncommercial surrogacy, we undermine some of our long-cherished values regarding family and society. One form this argument takes focuses on the notions of dignity and respect. As articulated in letter written by a Roman Catholic Monsignor and addressed to the task force, noncommercial surrogacy entails "disrespect for the person of the child and the birth mother. . . ." This line of argument also brings in the concept of "human dignity" in the Monsignor's statement that even noncommercial surrogacy is not "consistent with respect for human dignity."

Although some task force members accepted these arguments that noncommercial surrogacy is inherently immoral, others did not subscribe to the view that there are inherently unethical features of all surrogacy arrangements. For example, some objected to the contention that noncommercial surrogacy involves disrespect for family. In seeking to have a child to bring into their already existing family, a couple might be said to respect—rather than disrespect—family. The desire to bring a child into their family, and to love and nurture that child, appears to embody traditional family values rather than to contradict them.

Respect for the birth mother in noncommercial arrangements can be achieved by ensuring that she not be required to surrender a child she discovers she wants to keep, whether during her pregnancy or immediately after birth. The minutes of one task force meeting refer to the child "who is not valued as a unique individual but rather is treated as a commodity." However, in noncommercial surrogacy arrangements, the concept of "commodification" was held to be inapplicable. As for the other moral concept emphasized in the Monsignor's letter—"respect for human life and the dignity of the human person"—respect for the person of the child can be illustrated by the love and nurture that will be bestowed on it, either by the contracting parents who will rear the child or, in a failed surrogacy agreement, by the birth mother who has decided to keep the child.

A final line of argument focuses on the presumed consequences of permitting noncommercial surrogacy to exist. Since any ethical argument that appeals to the consequences of an act or practice must review the probable consequences of all reasonable alternative acts or practices, it is not sufficient to point only to the negative consequences that might result from allowing surrogacy arrangements to exist. It is necessary also to consider the consequences of prohibiting such arrangements.

The task force considered each set of possible or likely consequences: consequences for the child born of surrogacy arrangements, consequences for the birth mother, and consequences for "society." Those who supported the view that the negative consequences of noncommercial surrogacy arrangements warrant its prohibition were asked to spell out just what those probable consequences might be.

It proved difficult to argue, on empirical grounds, that the bad consequences for children born of surrogacy arrangements or for birth mothers who enter surrogacy agreements, or the vaguely imagined bad consequences for society, would outweigh the good consequences that could accrue for infertile couples seeking to make noncommercial surrogacy arrangements. Task force members on both sides of the debate agreed that the number of people likely to suffer ill effects is relatively small. The fact that only a small number of people would ever be affected reinforced the skepticism about the values of society being undermined if the state were to permit noncommercial surrogacy arrangements to exist.

The task force ultimately found the most compelling argument *against* prohibition of noncommercial surrogacy to lie in the limits of law in enforcing morality. Even when there is general agreement that a type of action or practice is morally wrong or ethically suspect, it does not automatically follow that the law should prohibit such acts or practices. Here it should be noted that not all task force members believe that noncommercial surrogacy arrangements are morally wrong or even questionable. One body of opinion holds that there is nothing inherently wrong with noncommercial surrogacy, despite the fact that bad consequences could flow from failed surrogacy agreements. Another view holds that there is something morally questionable about the practice of surrogacy in any form.

Yet even among those who maintained the latter position, a majority came to agree that worse consequences could flow from state prohibition of private arrangements within families or among friends than are likely to occur if noncommercial surrogacy is allowed to exist. These consequences include the prospect of state intrusion into the privacy of individuals and couples regarding their sexual and reproductive lives. It was noted, in particular, that a dangerous legal precedent could be set by restricting the reproductive freedom of couples to make private, noncommercial arrangements. State enforcement of such a ban could lead to intrusion into other reproductive areas, thus potentially compromising reproductive rights and liberties.

"Has everyone finished skimming these materials?" Maura O'Brien asks. "Good. Now will someone suggest wording for our recommendation regarding noncommercial surrogacy arrangements?"

Tod Nielsen volunteers. "How about this: The state should not legally prohibit noncommercial surrogacy arrangements."

"That sounds too permissive," Andrea Goldwoman argues. "It implies a tone of approval of the practice. We decided we wanted to discourage surrogacy, even in its noncommercial form."

"I agree," Father Timothy Reardon says. "The recommendation should sound as if the state discourages this immoral practice, even if it's not going to be legally prohibited."

Bill Ackerman suggests a different wording: "Any noncommercial surrogacy arrangement or any contractual provisions in association with a noncommercial surrogacy arrangement should be unenforceable."

"I don't think that quite captures the sense of moral disapproval we feel," Father Reardon says.

"Not everyone on this task force feels that sense of moral disapproval of noncommercial surrogacy, Father," Maura O'Brien admonishes. "Although we can't reach unanimity on the moral issue, I hope we can agree on wording for the policy recommendation. All in favor of Bill's suggestion, please signal by raising your hands. Good. All opposed?" Father Reardon's hand goes up. "Any abstentions?" Andrea Goldwoman raises her hand. "The proposed recommendation is approved," Maura says.

"Let's turn next to the question of whether there is a relevant distinction between the two forms of surrogacy with respect to a surrogate's claim on the child. I've asked Teddi Chernacoff to present an analysis that lays out the various options and moral arguments. We'll defer a vote on these options until our next meeting, but it would be useful to begin the discussion with a clear understanding of the different positions on this issue. Teddi, I'll turn it over to you."

Chernacoff begins: "When Maura asked me to make this presentation, she used the terms 'partial' and 'full' surrogacy to refer to the two different types of surrogate. I discovered that I had to look up those terms, to see how they were being used in the literature on surrogacy. Writers use 'partial' surrogacy to refer to a woman who is artificially inseminated and contributes her own egg to the pregnancy, and 'full' surrogacy for the situation using IVF and embryo transfer. According to this terminology, in full surrogacy the intended rearing parents are both genetically related to the child, since the husband's sperm is used to fertilize his wife's egg and the resulting embryo is implanted in the womb of the surrogate. So the 'full' surrogate is the gestational mother only. In partial surrogacy—the more common variety—sperm from the genetic father is used to inseminate the surrogate, who is both the genetic and the gestational mother. In this arrangement, the intended rearing mother is not genetically related to the child. Following this terminology—"

"Wait a second!" Tod Nielsen interrupts. "Are you telling us that the full surrogate is the gestational mother only? And the partial surrogate is both genetic and gestational mother? That terminology is not only confusing; it's counterintuitive!"

"That depends on what intuition you have," Chernacoff replies. "Look, it's possible for a woman to make either a gestational contribution, a genetic contribution, or both. Right? The gestational surrogate is called a 'full' surrogate because she might be considered a less 'real' mother than the partial surrogate, who contributes both necessary maternal elements to the creation of the child. A 'partial' surrogate is less a surrogate and more a real mother."

"I object to the term 'real mother,'" Andrea Goldwoman pipes up.

"As a matter of fact, so do I, as I'll be arguing in a moment," Chernacoff responds. "But first, can we clear up the confusion about partial and full surrogacy?"

"I still think it's counterintuitive," Nielsen insists. "With this crazy language, the 'partial' surrogate contributes more of herself, and is therefore more of a mother. The 'full' surrogate contributes less of herself, and is therefore less of a mother. Is this another case of 'less is more?' "

"I suggest we abandon the confusing terminology and adopt clear terms of our own that aren't counterintuitive," Bill Ackerman suggests. "Why don't we use the clearly understandable term 'gestational' for the surrogate who contributes only her womb? Then we have only to choose a word with clear meaning for the more common type of surrogate."

"Agreed. What should that word be?" Maura O'Brien asks.

"How about 'mother?' " Andrea Goldwoman suggests. "That's what she is, isn't she?"

"Strictly speaking, yes, but we do want the terminology we adopt for our report to be unequivocal. To call this type of surrogate the 'mother' is to fail to identify her as a surrogate."

"Right," says Goldwoman. "That's just the point."

"All right," Maura O'Brien interjects, "let's adopt a temporary solution for today's discussion, and the staff will propose some alternatives for our report. I suggest we use the term 'gestational surrogate' for the role Teddi has described as 'full' surrogate, and 'genetic/gestational surrogate' for the woman who makes both contributions. It's not elegant, but at least it's clear."

Chernacoff resumes her presentation. "It's often asked which criterion— genetic or gestational—should be used to determine who is the 'real' mother. I contend that this question is poorly formulated. Referring to the 'real' mother implies that it is a matter of *discovery*, rather than one calling for a *decision*. To speak of 'the real x' is to assume that there is an underlying metaphysical structure to be probed by philosophical inquiry. But now that medical technology has separated the two biological contributions to motherhood, in place of the single conjoint role provided by nature, some decisions will have to be made.

"One decision is conceptual, and a second is moral. The conceptual question is this: Should a woman whose contribution is only gestational be termed a 'mother' of the baby? By analogy with our concept of paternity, it makes sense to say that the woman who makes the genetic contribution in a surrogacy arrangement can properly be termed a 'mother' of the baby. So it must be decided whether there can be only one mother, conceptually speaking, or whether this technological advance calls for new terminology.

"Conceptual decisions often have implications beyond mere terminology. A decision *not* to use the term 'mother'—even when modified by the adjective 'gestational'—to refer to a woman who acts in this capacity can have important consequences for ethics and public policy. As a case in point, 'the Wayne County Circuit Court in Michigan issued an interim order declaring a gamete donor couple to be the biological parents of a fetus being carried to term by a woman hired to be the gestational mother. . . . Upon birth, the court entered an order that the names of the ovum and sperm donors be listed on the birth certificate, rather than that of the woman who gave birth, who was termed by the court a "human incubator.' "[7]

"The ethical question posed by the separation of biological motherhood into genetic and gestational components is this: Which role should entitle a woman to a greater claim on the baby, in case of dispute? Since the answer to this question cannot be reached by discovery but is, like the conceptual question, a matter for decision, we need to determine which factors are morally relevant and which have the greatest moral weight.

"The different possibilities I'm about to outline begin with the premise that surrogacy contracts are void and unenforceable. The task force has already agreed on that premise for our proposed policy. This means that no legal presumption is set up by the fact that there has been a prior contract between the surrogate and the intended rearing parents. If we accept the premise that a contractual provision to relinquish a child born of a surrogacy agreement has no legal force, we can turn to our central question: Is there a morally relevant distinction between the two forms of surrogacy with respect to a claim on the child? Who has the weightier moral claim when a surrogate is unwilling to give the baby up after its birth? Where should the moral presumption lie?

"Let me start with a frequently asked question: Who more deserves or has a 'right' to the child?[8] Three main views are outlined under this heading, each taking a different stance on which factor should be the criterion for the greater moral claim.

"The first view holds that gestation should be considered the overriding factor. Whether a woman is merely the gestational surrogate or also contributes her genetic material makes no difference in determining moral priorities; in either case, the surrogate is the primary mother because the criterion is gestation. One reason given in support of this presumption is 'the greater biological and psychological investment of the gestational mother in the child.'[9] This factor is sometimes referred to as 'sweat equity.' A related yet distinct reason is 'the biological reality that the [gestational] mother at this point has contributed more to the child's development, and that she will of necessity be present at birth and immediately thereafter to care for the child.'[10]

"The first of these two reasons focuses on what the gestational mother deserves, based on her investment in the child. The second reason, while mentioning her contribution, also focuses on the interests of the child during and immediately after birth.

"Now we come to the opposing view: namely, that genetics should be considered the overriding factor. In surrogacy arrangements, it is the inseminating male who is seen as the father, and not the husband of the woman who acts as a surrogate. This is because the genetic contribution is viewed as determinative for fatherhood. By analogy, the woman who makes the genetic contribution could be seen as the primary mother. This position sharply distinguishes between the claim to the child made by the two different types of surrogate. It makes the genetic/gestational surrogate the primary or even the sole mother. But now recall the fact that in artificial insemination by anonymous donor, the law recognizes the husband of the inseminated woman as the father. This shows that laws can be made to go either way.

"The court in *Smith & Smith v. Jones & Jones*—the Michigan case I cited earlier—relied on the analogy with paternity. The court said: 'The donor of the ovum, the biological mother, is to be deemed, in fact, the natural mother of this infant, as is the biological father to be deemed the natural father of this child.'[11]

"Legal precedents aside, is there a moral reason that could be invoked in support of this position? One possible reason is stated in terms of ownership of one's genetic products. Since each individual has a unique set of genes, people might be said to have a claim on what develops from their own genes, unless they have explicitly relinquished any such claims. This sense of 'ownership' reflects the felt desire to have genetically related children—the primary motivation behind all forms of assisted reproduction.

"Another possible reason for assigning greater weight to the genetic contribution is the child-centered position. Here it is argued that it is in children's best interest to be reared by parents to whom they are genetically related. As one contributor to the literature on surrogacy writes:

The most serious ethical problems in using third party donors in alternative reproduction concern the well-being of the potential child. . . . A child who has donor(s) intruded into its parentage will be cut off from its genetic heritage and part of its kinship relations in new ways. Even if there is no danger of transmitting unknown genetic disease or causing physiological harm to the child, the psychological relationship of the child to its parents is endangered—with or without the practice of deception and secrecy about its origins.[12]

"Additional considerations are often cited in support of this view about children. They derive from data concerning adopted children who have conducted searches for their biological parents, and similar experiences of children whose birth was a result of donor insemination and who have sought out their biological fathers. In gestational surrogacy the child is genetically related to both of the intended rearing parents. But it is too early for us to have any data on whether children born of gestational mothers might someday begin to seek out those women in a quest for their natural or 'real' mothers.

"Now a third view is a sort of hybrid between the two positions I've just discussed. This is the view that gestation and genetics both count in deciding who has the greater claim on a child in a disputed surrogacy arrangement. According to this position, the surrogate who contributes both egg and womb can better claim to be the primary mother than can the surrogate who contributes only her womb. Since the first type of surrogate makes both a genetic and a gestational contribution, in case of a dispute she gets to keep the baby instead of the biological father, who has made only one contribution. But this does not yet settle the question of who has a greater moral claim to the infant in cases where the gestational surrogate does not wish to give up the baby to the genetic parents. To determine that, greater weight must be given to either the gestational component or the genetic component.

"So far," Chernacoff continues, "I've been speaking only of the contributions of the surrogate for determining who has the greater moral claim to a child. This entirely ignores the contribution of the genetic father. Some people reject the idea that the only morally relevant determinants are the respective contributions of each type of surrogate. Their view rests on the biological conception of a family, and requires consideration of the genetic father. According to this position, two genetic contributions count more than none. So we have the following three subsidiary views.

"The first is that gestational surrogates have a lesser moral claim to the infant than the intended parents, both of whom have made a genetic contribution. This is because two (genetic) contributions count more than one (gestational) contribution. This view gives greatest weight to the concept of family based on genetic inheritance.

"Second is the view that a woman who contributes both egg and womb has a claim equal to that of the biological father, since both have made genetic contributions. If genetic contribution is what determines both 'true' motherhood and fatherhood, the policy implications of this view are that each case in which a genetic/gestational surrogate wishes to keep the baby would have to be settled in court in the manner of custody disputes. As a practical suggestion, this model is of little value. It throws every case of this type of surrogacy—the more common variety—open to such a dispute, which is to move backward in public policy regarding surrogacy.

"And finally, in this confusing array of possibilities, we have the view that genetic and gestational contributions should be given equal weight, and it is simply the number of contributions that counts. According to this position, the artificially inseminated surrogate has the greater moral claim, since she has made two contributions—genetic and gestational—while the father has made only one, the genetic contribution.

"I think this analysis includes the combinations of genetic and gestational contributions most likely to become considerations for assigning greater claims to a child in disputed surrogacy arrangements. I've refrained from drawing my own conclusions, since that's the job for the task force as a whole," Chernacoff concludes.

"Thank you, Teddi, that's very helpful. Let me review where we are at this point," Maura O'Brien says. "We have proposed a set of legal recommendations that should have the effect of discouraging all forms of surrogacy, especially the commercial variety. We would prohibit financial payments, other than for medical expenses, to women who serve as surrogates. We would ban all commercial brokers or intermediaries outright, suggesting that the state legislature assign criminal penalties. And we have decided that all contracts in which surrogates promise to relinquish custody or to terminate their parental rights at birth should be void and legally unenforceable. Even with these discouraging features, it is entirely possible that some people will choose to enter surrogacy arrangements anyway, and take their chances. So we still need to arrive at policy guidelines that cover situations in which children are born through surrogacy and the birth mother decides she wants to keep the child. And drawing on the presentation we just heard from Teddi, we have to address the question of whether a claim made by the intended rearing parents, where both are genetic parents of the child, should be viewed differently from cases in which only the father is genetically related to the child. In view of the lateness of the hour, I suggest we defer these topics to next month's meeting, when we'll complete our deliberations for the final report."

Bonnie rushes to Robbie's bedroom to look at her sleeping baby as soon as she gets home. After stroking his back and kissing him, she joins Larry in the living room.

"I'm scared, Larry, petrified at what could happen. You wouldn't believe what I heard tonight at that meeting. This task force has decided that commercial surrogacy arrangements should be illegal. They even talked about criminal penalties!"

"Who would get these penalties? The parents? The surrogate?"

"They didn't go into detail at the meeting. They said it would be left to the state legislature to decide. But it sounded like they were talking about the surrogate, the parents, and brokers like the Fecundity Center."

"No wonder the clinic decided to get out of the surrogacy business so fast. Jeez! That would make us criminals!"

"I know, and that seems wrong to me. The task force is supposed to be talking about the ethics of surrogacy. I don't think it's ethical to make people like us criminals, just because we wanted so badly to have a baby."

"Don't worry, Bon, they can't make laws like this retroactive. I'm sure it could only apply in the future."

"Yes, but I still don't think that's right. It would make other people like us criminals if they decided to do what we did."

"Did they say anything about the surrogate mother having custody of the baby?"

"More bad news. They left the details to next month's meeting, but as I understood the recommendations they've already agreed on, surrogates would have the right to keep the baby if they wanted to."

"I can't believe it. In all cases?"

"Well, they are going to discuss gestational surrogacy, in particular, next time. But look at this handout, with their recommendations. They voted to approve these three at an earlier meeting."

Larry reads the sheet Bonnie hands to him, recommending that all surrogacy contracts be held void and unenforceable, and that commercial arrangements be made illegal and subject to civil or criminal penalties.

Bonnie adds: "When they say it's unenforceable, it means that even if a surrogate signs a contract saying she'll give up the baby, there's no way to enforce the contract. We couldn't go to court and ask them to make Gloria give us Robbie if she decided in the hospital she wanted to keep him."

"What about now? Once we have the baby? Is there any way Gloria could get him back?"

"Oh, Larry, I don't know. Next month they're going to talk about things like that."

"The longer it takes them, the better it'll be for us. Nobody in his right mind will take a baby away from the parents who love it and care for it properly."

"I hope you're right. I don't know if they're going to discuss visitation rights, but I'm definitely going again next month."

"Let's get a babysitter so I can go too," Larry says. "I only hope Gloria doesn't find out about this task force. It might put some new ideas in her head, and we've got enough to worry about already."

Reaching Closure

       Teddi Chernacoff is lurching from one meeting to the next. On the same day, the hospital ethics committee is scheduled in the afternoon and the Task Force on Reproduction in the evening. Following a medical school seminar in which she makes a presentation on physician-assisted suicide, Chernacoff rushes into the ethics committee meeting. She catches her breath and switches bioethical gears from death to birth.

Dr. Becker calls on Evan to present the polished version of the hurriedly drafted statement on forced cesarean sections he proposed at the previous month's meeting.

"Well, this may surprise you, but after giving the matter some thought, I hereby retract my statement."

"Why? It sounded good to me," one physician says.

"Good! I knew you'd see the ethical and legal merits of the ACOG committee opinion," Chernacoff says, gloating.

"Remind us. What were the recommendations of the American College of Obstetricians and Gynecologists?" Dr. Becker asks.

"Simply that 'every reasonable effort should be made to protect the fetus, but the pregnant woman's autonomy should be respected,' that 'the use of the courts to resolve these conflicts is almost never warranted,' and that 'the use of judicial authority to implement treatment regimens in order to protect the fetus violates the pregnant woman's autonomy' and may lead to 'the criminalization of noncompliance with medical recommendations.' If that statement was found appropriate for the nation's obstetricians and gynecologists, it should be good enough for us," Chernacoff asserts.

"Before we go back to the ACOG statement, can we first hear why Evan wants to retract his prepared statement?"

"My reason is simple," Evan answers. "Policies ought to help direct action. This one fails to do so; it amounts to having no policy at all. This statement is useless to clinicians. As an alternative to a wishy-washy policy devoid of guidance, I think we as an ethics committee have the option of issuing a white paper pointing out various specific approaches to the problem and outlining competing arguments."

"Does anyone have any suggestions?" Dr. Becker asks the committee.

"Yes, let's drop the whole thing," one member replies. "If we can't reach agreement, we can't have a policy. It's as simple as that."

After a moment's silence, Evan asks for the floor. "When I became unhappy with our nonpolicy, I did a bit of research. Remember the case that occurred in Washington, D.C., a few years ago? The one in which a hospital obtained a court order to perform a cesarean section on a pregnant woman dying of cancer?"

Several committee members nod. Someone else asks, "Could you remind us of the details?"

"Not all the details are important for our purposes, but basically what happened was that the patient, a woman named Angela Carder, had a recurrence of an earlier cancer; during her remission from the cancer, however, she had intentionally become pregnant and had actually completed about twenty-six weeks of her pregnancy. As her condition rapidly deteriorated, it became difficult to communicate with her, and when her doctors asked her if she still wanted to have the baby, her reply was unclear. She seemed to be refusing a cesarean section, but her precise wishes could not really be known. The hospital decided to go to court for a ruling on what was legally required, and—"

"That's exactly what I would have done," the hospital administrator interjects. "Cases involving a fetus are legal matters, and neither the patient nor the physicians may decide—"

"Bob, I'm going to rule you out of order. Let Evan finish," Dr. Becker reprimands.

"Okay, yes, so the hospital's general counsel got in touch with a judge, who decided to hold a hearing in the hospital. I should add that the patient's husband and her parents were in the hospital at the time, and both stood by Angela. Not only that, but Angela's own physician was willing to go along with her apparent wishes not to have the cesarean performed. Anyway, to cut this short, the judge did order the C-section. A baby girl was delivered and died within two and a half hours. Angela Carder herself died two days later."

"What a tragic story," a social worker laments.

"It was an outrage," Teddi Chernacoff exclaims.

"I still say the hospital did what it had to do," the administrator asserts. "If you want to blame anyone, it should be the judge."

"Well, you might blame that judge, but let me tell you the sequel," Evan resumes. "The District of Columbia Court of Appeals made a later ruling on the case and vacated the order. That's legal jargon for saying that the original court order would not stand as a precedent, although of course the circumstances could not be reversed. The appellate court stated that 'it would be far better if judges were not called to patients' bedsides and required to made quick decisions on issues of life and death.' "[1]

"Well, that's very interesting," a physician muses, "but how does it apply to us?"

"Strictly speaking, it doesn't," Evan replies. "We're not in that jurisdiction, and a court in our own district could conceivably rule differently. But what I really want to bring to your attention is the policy later adopted by the hospital. The Court of Appeals ruling wasn't the final legal action in the Carder case. The American Civil Liberties Union filed a separate malpractice and civil rights case against the George Washington University Medical Center for its treatment of Angela Carder and for its decision to involve the court. As a result of the settlement, the medical center developed a policy on decision-making by pregnant patients that now serves as a model for other hospitals to emulate. I've brought along copies of the policy so you can see how one hospital resolved to handle these issues. Let me walk you through the document and call your attention to some of the highlights.

"First, the policy states: 'We base our policies regarding decision-making on this hospital's (and the medical profession's) strong commitment to respecting the autonomy of all patients with capacity.'[2] It adds that respect for autonomy does not end just because a patient refuses a course of action that physicians recommend. Moreover, the same ethical, legal, and medical standards that apply to nonpregnant patients apply equally to the decision-making process with a pregnant patient. The policy emphasizes the importance of counseling pregnant women and also urges that when a pregnant patient's decision 'appears unnecessarily to disserve her own or fetal welfare, great care should be taken to verify that her decision is both informed and authentic.'[3] When such circumstances arise, the physician should seek to explore the reasons that lie behind the patient's decision.

"Nevertheless, if all counseling and explorations with the patient fail, the ultimate decision is left to the woman. The policy states: 'When a fully informed and competent pregnant patient persists in a decision which may disserve her own or fetal welfare, this hospital's policy is to accede to the pregnant patient's preference whenever possible.' The policy also addresses the issue of pregnant patients who are not capable of consenting to or refusing treatment in an informed fashion. In such cases, the document recognizes the authority of a proxy for the patient, building in appropriate safeguards to protect the welfare of the patient and the fetus. The policy states that 'the hospital will accede to a well-founded surrogate's decision whenever possible.'[4]

"Finally, and significantly, this model policy asserts that courts are an inappropriate forum for resolving ethical issues. It endorses a strong commitment to keeping health care decision-making within the patient-physician relationship. The policy concludes with the statement: 'It will rarely be appropriate to seek judicial intervention to assess or override a pregnant patient's decision.'[5]

"I move that we adopt the same policy in this hospital," Chernacoff says.

One physician remarks: "I hate to say it, but I think the policy of George Washington University Hospital is a result of the bad publicity the hospital received, and the fact that the District of Columbia Court of Appeals reversed the lower court's decision."

"So what if that's true?" Chernacoff replies. "The motives need not have anything to do with the morality of the action. If the policy is ethically sound, the justification lies in the values it seeks to uphold, not in the causes that led to its adoption."

After lengthy deliberation the ethics committee approves the policy, with only two abstentions and no votes against. Dr. Becker adjourns the committee, thanking the members for their endurance.

❁

Chernacoff leaves the hospital ethics committee meeting at 6:00 P.M. and gets into her car for the forty-minute drive to the state capital, where the Task Force on Reproduction meets. She arrives just as the members are finishing a buffet supper. "If I see another cold cut, I'm going to scream," Chernacoff confides to Tod Nielsen.

"Would you rather poached salmon with crème fraiche?" Nielsen asks.

"That would be nice, but fat chance!" Chernacoff retorts. She grabs an iced tea just as the chair is calling the task force to order. As she takes her seat, she notices Bonnie and Larry Roberts sitting in a back row with several other observers.

Maura O'Brien begins. "Recall that we have two main issues to resolve at today's meeting. Both have to do with policy guidelines to cover situations in which children are born through surrogacy and the birth mother decides she wants to keep the child. The first is to reach some consensus on the question of whether a claim made by the intended rearing parents, when both are genetic parents of the child, should be viewed differently from cases in which only the father is genetically related to the child. To put it another way, should a surrogate who is only the gestational mother have the same rights as the surrogate who is both the genetic and gestational mother? Teddi gave us a detailed analysis at last month's meeting but refrained from drawing a conclusion. The second issue relates to visitation rights of noncustodial parents. That is, after a surrogacy dispute has been settled by law or decided by a court, and custody is awarded to one parent or a couple, should the noncustodial parent have visitation rights? Let's hear first from Bill Ackerman, who has a legal update on some court rulings."

"Thanks Maura. I'm not going to deal with cases in which the court had to decide whether surrogacy arrangements violate state adoption laws,[6] since we've already determined that our policy recommendations would prohibit commercial surrogacy and include the same provisions found in adoption policies regarding a waiting period after the birth of the baby and the right of the birth mother to change her mind. But one recent case from California is on point regarding gestational surrogacy. This is *Anna J. v. Mark C.*[7]

"In this case, a married couple, Mark and Crispina Calvert, made a surrogacy agreement with Anna Johnson, a co-worker of Ms. Calvert. Crispina Calvert had had a partial hysterectomy but could still produce eggs. So an embryo produced by Mark Calvert's sperm and his wife's egg was implanted in Anna Johnson, who agreed that she would relinquish all parental rights to the child in return for $10,000, to be paid in installments. After the initial agreement was made, relations between the two sides deteriorated. Anna had not disclosed to the Calverts the fact that she had previously suffered several stillbirths and miscarriages. And for her part, Anna was upset because she claimed that the couple had abandoned her during an onset of premature labor. Apparently, there were also some disputes about money. Anna Johnson claimed that the Calverts did not do enough to obtain a life insurance policy for her that they had agreed to as part of their contract.

"I think those aspects of the case are irrelevant to our concerns. The bottom line is that Anna Johnson filed an action to be declared the mother of the child, and the trial court decided in favor of Mark and Crispina, ruling that they were the child's 'genetic, biological and natural' father and mother. There had been a court order allowing Anna to visit the child until the trial, but the trial court also ruled that Anna Johnson had no 'parental' rights to the child and that the contract was legal and enforceable against Anna's claims. The California Court of Appeals affirmed the lower court's decision. Under a provision of the California Parentage Act, the court found that Crispina Calvert was the 'natural' mother of the child and Mark Calvert was not precluded from being the legal father.[8] As courts usually do, the California appellate court called for legislative action in the matter of surrogacy agreements."

"Thank you, Bill. Your last remark about the court calling for the legislature to do something reminds us why we're here. The New Jersey Supreme Court in the Baby M case in 1988 also called for the state legislature to take action, but as we know, the New Jersey state legislature still has not enacted legislation dealing with surrogacy."[9]

"I think this case shows us just what's wrong with terms like 'natural' when they're used to describe what counts as a mother," Teddi Chernacoff says. "The woman who gives birth and the woman who contributes the egg can both be said to be 'natural' mothers. It's our job to determine which woman should be presumed to have custody in case the surrogate is unwilling to give up the child."

"I'm confused," says Jeanne Lodge, the community representative. "I thought we'd already decided that surrogacy should be prohibited and that surrogacy contracts should be unenforceable. How come we're still talking about who should get the baby?"

"Didn't you ever hear of people breaking laws?" asks Vera Rodriguez, the nurse.

"Let me remind us where we are on this," interjects Maura O'Brien. "We did decide that commercial surrogacy should be legally prohibited, and also that all surrogacy contracts should be unenforceable. But those conclusions don't yet give guidance in cases where people do break the law or make noncommercial contracts. In our recommendations we could leave everything up to the courts to decide, on the assumption that if people do go through with surrogacy arrangements and end up in dispute, they will take the case to court. Or we could build into our recommendations to the legislature the provisions we think the law ought to have."

"I see now," says Jeanne Lodge.

"We're open for discussion," O'Brien resumes.

"Is there any psychological data that can help us out here?" asks LeRoy Johnson, the state assemblyman. "I think the legislature would like to be sure that any laws we pass are on sound footing."

"There is literature on maternal-infant bonding," volunteers Anthony Romano, the ob-gyn on the task force. "Whether or not birth mothers are genetically related to their children, they develop emotional attachments to their babies in utero."

"Are there data on that?" inquires LeRoy Johnson.

"As a matter of fact, there are," Dr. Romano replies. "Mothers develop good feelings toward their unborn children because of fetal movements, which have 'a major effect on a mother's thoughts or feelings about the baby. The mother often begins to feel the baby is hers.' And one study that tested newborns' ability to detect their mothers' voices 'showed that 15 out of 16 babies triggered recordings of their mothers' reading stories that were read to them while in the womb by sucking on rubber nipples. On the third day of life, the baby will suck to hear the story he heard in utero.' "[10]

"That sounds incredible to me," Tod Nielsen ventures.

"Incredible or not, that's what the study shows."

"What about the women? I'd like to hear more about them," Andrea Goldwoman insists.

Roberta Bernstein, the psychologist, speaks up. "I haven't said much throughout our deliberations. That's because I really don't think there's much in the way of hard data for these theories about maternal-infant bonding. With all due respect to the studies Dr. Romano cited, I question whether the literature on 'bonding' and other studies of women who give up their children for adoption are appropriate for our purpose. The meaning of the concept of bonding is imprecise.[11] Sometimes it's used simply as a synonym for the word 'attachment,' yet the two have different meanings. 'Bonding' refers to the mother's response to the infant, and 'attachment' refers to the slowly developing emotional connection between the infant and a caretaker who is sensitive to the child's needs. Both the pediatric and popular literature would lead us to believe that 'bonding' benefits the people who will care for the infant by making them more responsive to the baby than caregivers who have not had that experience. But I must repeat that studies of the value of bonding for infants or mothers have been questioned on a number of different grounds. There remains a question whether the long-term benefits to mothers or their children that were originally claimed to result from bonding have been demonstrated. But having said that," Roberta Bernstein continues," I want to tip my hand in favor of granting custody to the birth mother, whether she is the genetic mother also or has simply served as a gestational surrogate."

"Maura, can we go back to something we discussed at an earlier meeting?" asks John Ward, the Methodist pastor. "I can't help thinking about the similarities and differences between surrogacy and egg donation. In cases of egg donation, it's always assumed that the woman who donates eggs to an infertile couple is *not* the mother of the child. Yet by the criteria used in the California case, an egg donor, as the genetic mother, would have to be the 'natural' mother. Where does that leave us?"

"That's not quite accurate," Bill Ackerman interrupts. "The court found that Crispina Calvert was the 'natural' mother of the child under a provision of the California Parentage Act. That doesn't apply to this situation."

"But wait, maybe John has a point here," Tod Nielsen interjects. "Maybe we should strive for consistency between surrogacy arrangements and egg donation situations. A birth mother is a birth mother is a birth mother—"

"That reminds me," says Vera Rodriguez. "Remember the two Australian cases we heard about at an earlier meeting? Linda Kirkman was the gestational mother of a baby conceived with her sister's egg and destined to live with the infertile sister and her husband. Linda Kirkman said, 'I always considered myself her aunt.' Then there was Carol Chan, who donated eggs so that her sister Susie could bear and raise a child. Carol

Chan said: 'I could never regard the twins as anything but my nephews.' These two births occurred in Melbourne, Australia, within two weeks of each other.[12] In one case the genetic mother got the child, and in the other case the gestational mother got the child. Where does that leave us?"

"But remember, Vera, these two sisters were happy with the arrangements they had made. There was no dispute over the child," Teddi Chernacoff points out. "It's reasonable to assume that such arrangements between sisters are true examples of 'altruistic' surrogacy or egg donation: that is, without expectation of personal gain. At the same time, these 'altruistic' sisters are most likely not acting merely as a means to the ends of others. Sisters who love each other feel pained by the other's loss or adversity, so they serve their own emotional ends as well as the ends of their sisters by assisting in a reproductive arrangement."

"Well, there's still the possibility of familial problems down the road," Roberta Bernstein points out. "Linda and Carol may feel like aunts at the time of gestation and birth. But what happens when their sisters' babies grow older? Carol Chan's 'nephews' are her genetic sons, so they may resemble her physically or behaviorally more than they resemble their gestational and adoptive mother. Or, if Linda Kirkman's "niece" is informed that she was carried in utero by Linda rather than by her genetic and adoptive mother, she may feel a bond with the woman who gestated her."

"Yes, but there's no way to predict what thoughts or feelings may ensue, and also no way to judge whether any thoughts or feelings are unjustified in these novel family situations," Anthony Romano says. "Just because they're novel and unpredictable does not make them morally suspect."

"Spoken like a true philosopher," Chernacoff asserts.

"But who says these children have to be told anything about their origins?" LeRoy Johnson asks. "Isn't that opening a can of worms?"

"Are you suggesting the parents ought to lie to these children?"

"Which parents? The genetic mother? The gestational mother? The intended rearing parents? The sperm-donating father? The adoptive parents?"

"Order! Order!" Maura O'Brien yells. "I recognize Roberta Bernstein."

"You know, considerable experience with adoption and artificial insemination demonstrates that 'family secrets' can often be very destructive. 'When a parent reveals a secret or, even more important, a lie, a basic trust is broken. Childhood memories are rewritten.'"[13]

"What are you suggesting, Roberta?"

"I'm suggesting that parents cannot pretend that children born of a gestational surrogate have no origins outside themselves. The life of these children begins when they are in the womb, inside the gestational mother. This is part of the child's history, part of the child's biography. Children in this situation have three parents, and that ought to be acknowledged." [14]

"We seem to be moving toward a consensus here," Maura O'Brien observes. "Any further thoughts?"

"Yes," Andrea Goldwoman says. "My view is that the process of gestation and the act of giving birth clearly weigh more heavily in determining who has the greater claim on a child in cases of dispute. I think the same criterion should be used in surrogacy as in egg donation for identifying the woman who should be able to make all determinations: the woman who gestates and gives birth to the child."

"Anyone disagree?"

"I'm still uncertain," Tod Nielsen says tentatively. "Remember, a few meetings ago I gave a presentation about procreative liberty and constitutional rights. Well, there's a long tradition in law about genetic inheritance and the presumptions in favor of genetic parentage. It's hard for me to shed those presumptions."

Bill Ackerman speaks up: "That's all true, Tod, but surely you're not forgetting the uniformity of laws on artificial insemination: the husband of the woman who is inseminated is, by legal convention, held to be the father of the child once he agrees to the insemination. Laws can be made to go the way we want them to. Gestational surrogacy is a novel arrangement, and we are in a position to recommend the best solution, from the point of view of public policy."

"And ethics," Chernacoff adds.

"I think we're losing sight of the importance of family," Jeanne Lodge ventures. "Laws and public policy should be made for people. Don't we have an obligation to promote what's good for families?"

"Sure," Bill Ackerman responds, "but it all depends on what you mean by family."

"Families are genetically related individuals and those brought together in the sacrament of marriage," Father Reardon asserts. "Is there any other meaning?"

"That's just too simple," Andrea Goldwoman says. "I know of a gay couple who decided to solidify their relationship by taking matrimonial vows. Despite the fact that their marriage is not recognized by civil law, they found an ordained minister who was willing to perform the marriage ceremony. They are now a married couple, a family. Later they applied to be foster parents of children with AIDS whose biological parents had died or abandoned them. The foster agency accepted the couple, and the children were placed in their foster care. They are now a family.

"In another case I know of, a judge in New York City approved the adoption of a six-year-old boy by the lesbian partner of the child's biological mother.[15] The biological mother had been artificially inseminated in 1985. In her ruling, the Surrogate Court judge said, 'No provision of New York law requires that the adoptive parent be of any particular gender.' The judge added that the decision conferred 'legal recognition of their mutual status as parents,' despite the absence of a marriage certificate. The three are now a family, with one parent genetically related to the child and the other a nonrelated, adoptive parent of the same sex."

Father Reardon tries to speak but is interrupted by LeRoy Johnson. "You know, I think being a family is a matter of how people consider each other. I know a woman who referred to her 'brother' for years. One day I said to her, 'I never knew you had a brother. I thought you told me you were an only child.' She replied, 'Well, we're not really related; we just grew up together. He wasn't officially adopted into my family, but we grew up thinking of each other as brother and sister and always refer to each other that way.'"

"Here's another one," John Ward volunteers. "I was counseling a young unmarried couple who had a child and decided not to marry. When the boy was very young, he was legally adopted by his biological father's sister and her husband. Although the boy was told he was adopted, his adoptive parents never informed him that his uncle (whom he knew) was really his father or that his adoptive mother was really his biological aunt. Out of respect for the wishes of the boy's biological father, that information was kept secret. Another family member with whom the boy was close was an aunt, the sister of both his biological father and his adoptive mother. The boy had the same genetic relationship to this aunt as he did to his adoptive mother."

"Too much!"

"Could you go through that one again, John?"

"What are all these examples supposed to show?" asks the exasperated Father Reardon. "That a family can be anything you want it to be? That's a perversion of language, custom, and sacred covenants."

"With all due respect, Father Reardon, that view is narrowly ethnocentric. Different cultures have different definitions of what counts as a family," Roberta Bernstein points out.

"Not only that, but language is always changing, adapting to new developments," Teddi Chernacoff asserts. "Here's a definition of 'family' I came across recently in a journal. This definition was introduced to take account of changing psychosocial circumstances in an era of AIDS: 'Family members are individuals who by birth, adoption, marriage, or declared commitment share deep personal connections and are mutually entitled to receive and obligated to provide support of various kinds to the extent possible, especially in times of need.' " [16]

"I think we've spent enough time on this discussion. Let's move on," Maura O'Brien urges. "We need to come to some resolution on the question of whether gestational surrogates should be treated just like surrogates who are both gestational and genetic mothers."

Tod Nielsen takes the floor. "I'd like to propose that we agree to a presumption favoring the birth mother, whether she's the genetic mother or not, in cases of disputed surrogacy arrangements. That presumption would further a number of public policy objectives." He reads from his notes:

First, a birth mother presumption recognizes that the experience of pregnancy constitutes a substantial physiological (and potentially psychosocial) involvement of the birth mother with the child. In this respect it is consistent with a broadly shared view of the birth mother as the "natural" mother and the parent closest to the child at the time of birth. Second, a birth mother presumption significantly lessens the potential for a highly visible and destructive class and economic bias that is present in a litigation process, and substantially redresses the imbalance in bargaining power that is generally present between the . . . "surrogate" and the natural father. Third, a birth mother preference rule encourages parties to resolve their disputes without resorting to litigation, a result that benefits society, the custodial parent(s), and the child.[17]

"Very eloquent, Tod."

"Yes, it captures the consensus we've been moving toward."

"I move that we adopt Tod's proposal."

"Second the motion."

"Anyone opposed?" Maura O'Brien asks. No objections are raised. "Good. Tod, would you please write that wording up for us so we can incorporate it into our justification in our written recommendations? Thanks. Now we agreed to discuss one more issue at tonight's meeting: the question of visitation rights for the noncustodial parent in cases of disputed surrogacy agreements. Who wants to start?"

Bill Ackerman responds. "Well, we can begin by noting that in the Baby M case the judge granted visitation rights to Mary Beth Whitehead, and in the California case we just heard about the Court of Appeal denied visitation rights. Should it make any difference whether the surrogate was both the genetic and gestational mother, like Mary Beth Whitehead, or the gestational mother only, like Anna Johnson? I think not."

"I agree," says Chernacoff. "Once we've determined that it's gestation and birth that really matter, there's no further ground for distinguishing between the two forms of surrogacy."

"How does the possibility of granting visitation rights to the noncustodial parent square with adoption laws and practices?" John Ward asks.

"This public policy solution is not modeled after adoption laws. In that situation, a birth mother is given the opportunity to change her mind about a prearranged adoption plan, but once she gives up her initial right to the child and after a legally determined waiting period, she retains no visitation rights. Our policy on surrogacy is more like divorce settlements that involve custody arrangements. Even when sole custody is awarded to one parent, the noncustodial parent is usually granted visitation rights," Ackerman says.

"You mean surrogacy is like divorce?"

"Don't be facetious. We're talking about models of custody arrangements."

"How can we know what's in the child's best interest? Should the 'best interest of the child' be the overriding concern in such arrangements? And what about the interests of the noncustodial parents?" asks Jeanne Lodge.

Roberta Bernstein tries to respond. "I believe it will be difficult, if not impossible, in most cases of disputed surrogacy arrangements to determine whether visitation would be in the best interests of the child. The doctrine of the 'best interest of the child' is brought in to ensure that a public policy in this area will be sufficiently child-centered, and not based solely on the wishes of the biological or gestational parents. That seems right to me. Yet it seems hopeless to seek to determine, on a case-by-case basis at the time of birth or even some time later, whether granting visitation rights to the noncustodial parent would be in the best interest of the child. In most cases, there could hardly be enough factual information for anyone to make a decision on that basis."

Father Reardon has been silent for a long time. "How could it *not* be in children's interest to maintain contact with their biological parents? Don't we have many reported experiences of adopted children and children who learned that their birth resulted from artificial insemination who then embarked on a search for their biological parents? Having contact with biological parents is an important value, one that should be upheld.

Although I still think that surrogacy in any form is wrong, we have to admit that these things will happen. I think we have no alternative but to recommend the possibility of visitation rights for the noncustodial parent."

"Any legal cases you know of, Tod or Bill?"

"Well yes, there's one in California—"

"As usual!"

"But," Bill Ackerman continues, "as usual there are special features of the particular case. A child was born to a preschool teacher, Nancy Barrass, who was inseminated with the sperm of Timothy Myers. The intended rearing parents, according to the contract, were Mr. Myers and his wife, Charlotte. Nancy Barrass's lawyer argued that her client, surrounded by people interested in depriving her of her parental rights, had not understood that in signing the agreement she was giving up all rights to see her child again. The problem with this case was that the boy was nearly five years old at the time the appeal was being made. The lawyer for Nancy Barrass contended that it's not detrimental to a child to have two mothers. The deputy attorney general, however, noted that social workers and a psychologist who had studied and carefully interviewed both the Myers couple and Barrass had issued a 'very strong report' recommending that the child go to the Myerses and asserting that a 'competitive parenting situation would result' if Barrass were allowed to share in raising the child. Barrass's lawyer said that if the usual adoption procedures had been used, there would have been adequate counseling so the woman would have known what she was signing.[18] The case is now on appeal, so I guess it doesn't help us much."

"So you see, in that case the surrogate was both the gestational and the genetic mother, and still the judge did not grant her visitation rights. But in the other California case, the argument was that Anna Johnson was not the mother because she was only the gestational surrogate. I guess I still don't get it," laments LeRoy Johnson.

"Let's forget about what all these judges are saying and decide what we think is right!" Teddi Chernacoff exclaims. "I must confess, I'm ambivalent and uncertain about granting visitation rights to noncustodial parents when surrogacy arrangements do not work out as planned. I think it's because of the profound difficulty of weighing that value, having contact with one's biological parents, against competing considerations. There's the possibility of divergent views on child rearing between the custodial and noncustodial parents; the prospect of residual hostility between these parties; the disruptions in a child's social and emotional life caused by the circumstances of visitation, and so on. If anything is likely to disrupt a family, granting visitation rights to noncustodial parents in disputed surrogacy arrangements fits the bill. Yet by default, it may turn out to be the least harmful solution when things don't work out as planned."

"Well," says Maura O'Brien," we don't seem to be making any headway. We've seen that judges have decided different things in different cases. And I wish there was more in the way of psychological data. Roberta, do you have any further thoughts?"

"I'm afraid I can't be of any more help on this. 'Some experts in child psychology argue that the child's interests are best served by allowing him or her the opportunity to maintain contact with all biological parents; others maintain that it may be disruptive and confusing to the child to have that contact, especially if it is contrary to the wishes of the custodial parent.' " [19]

"So much for psychological experts!" sighs LeRoy Johnson.

"I think we really only have one recourse," Chernacoff suggests. "That's to 'recognize that a child may have competing interests in psychological stability and in maintaining contact with his or her biological parents. Both interests should be considered.' " [20]

"Okay, then, here's some proposed wording," Bill Ackerman offers. He reads the following statement:

A presumption should be established in favor of visitation rights for the noncustodial parent, unless it is demonstrated that such visitation would be contrary to the best interests of the child. The extent and conditions of visitation should be considered on a case-by-case basis, with due regard for the child's interests both in psychological stability and in the maintenance of contact with the child's biological parents. [21]

"Fine," Maura O'Brien says. "I think that's enough for this evening. "We'll send you written versions of all the proposals discussed tonight before the next meeting. Thanks again for all your hard work. See you next month."

As they drive away from the task force meeting, Larry is irritated. "You know," he says to Bonnie, "it's not fair. We tried to adopt a baby, and the agency didn't find us 'suitable.' But now we hear that some judge allows a couple of lesbians to adopt. How come we weren't suitable and they were?"

"I think you're prejudiced," Bonnie replies. "You're forgetting that one of the lesbians was the natural mother of the baby. The judge just let her partner adopt. Anyway, that's none of our business." Then, hesitantly: "Larry, after what we heard, maybe it wouldn't be such a bad thing if Gloria got to see little Robbie. It was interesting to hear about those Australian sisters. The one who was the surrogate and the one who donated her eggs both said they felt like aunts to their sister's children."

"Well of course!" Larry sputters. They were *sisters*. Gloria isn't your sister or mine!" He becomes thoughtful as his comment makes him remember Frannie. "I've been thinking of something else, though, Bon. It's the thing we've gone round and round on—whether we should keep it a secret or tell him that he had a surrogate mother. We haven't talked about that lately, but we really should think about what's right."

"If we tell, then won't he want to know who the surrogate mother was?"

"Not necessarily," Larry says. "We're his genetic parents, and that's what counts most. When adopted children go on searches for their real parents, isn't it because they want to know about their genes? Robbie will know, so why should he care if a surrogate carried him in the womb for nine months?"

"Well, we just don't know. But the women I spoke to at Resolve said they're going to keep it a secret."

"Right now we still have Gloria to worry about. Once we get her out of the picture, we can decide about these other things."

"Larry, if she gets to visit Robbie, *she* might tell him. Wouldn't it be better if it comes from us?"

"That's for sure! All the more reason not to give in to her."

The couple is silent the rest of the way home.

❧

Several days later Gloria Gardner telephones. She asks to come over for a talk, and Larry and Bonnie have no choice but to agree. They arrange for her to come on Saturday during Robbie's afternoon nap.

The three parents settle themselves awkwardly in the Robertses' living room. Gloria begins: "I'll get right to the point. I read in the paper what the Task Force on Reproduction recommended. I think I'm on good ground now, and I'm planning to fight for visitation rights."

Larry points out that there's no law in their state about surrogate visitation rights.

"I know that, but my lawyer will have a pretty good case with the task force recommendations on my side," Gloria responds.

"That may be true," Bonnie says, "but our lawyer will defend our rights."

"Yes, and he'll bring up the Anna Johnson case in California," Larry adds. "That didn't turn out so good for the surrogate. She was a gestational surrogate, just like you," Larry says, a bit smugly.

"But that was in California," Gloria says, "and they didn't have the task force recommendations to back them up. By the time we get to court, my lawyer thinks there may be a law—but look, do we really want to spend a lot of money on lawyers? And what about all the publicity? Do we want to deal with that?"

Bonnie and Larry glance at one another. The last thing they want is publicity. Bonnie recalls seeing a newspaper article after the Baby M case, with the headline "And What about Baby M's Ruined Life?"[22] Larry wonders how anything could ever be kept secret from Robbie if there are court cases that drag on, newspaper clippings in somebody's scrapbook, or worse. What if Gloria decides to sell her story to a paperback writer? Or to a TV producer for a docudrama? Someone is bound to want to cash in on a story like this.

Bonnie asks tentatively, "Gloria, suppose we do let you visit Robbie. What are you going to tell him? Who should we say you are?"

"I've thought about that," Gloria replies. "You probably already named a godmother for Robbie, but when I was a kid my parents had close friends we called 'uncle' and 'aunt.' Couldn't I be 'Aunt Gloria'?"

"My brother's wife is his aunt," Larry snaps. Then, to his own surprise, he adds: "I had a sister, but she died."

"I'm sorry," Gloria says with some feeling. "I'm really sorry."

"Poor Frannie," Bonnie explains. "It's only been a few months since she died."

"Frannie? I had a good friend in high school named Frannie Roberts."

"What year did you graduate?" Larry asks.

When Gloria's answer confirms that she and Frannie had indeed been high school friends, Larry's attitude changes. Thinking of his sister, the aunt his little boy will never know, he says thoughtfully, "Maybe it would be good for Robbie to have an aunt."

"I promise you, I'll never tell Robbie what I did. Now that I know Frannie Roberts was your sister, I feel like we're friends. I never wanted this to become a legal battle."

"I'm relieved too," Bonnie says. "I'm so glad we won't have to deal with lawyers and judges and court orders."

They spend the rest of the afternoon talking about Frannie, Gloria recalling the good times they had in high school, the experiences and confidences they shared. Bonnie turns abruptly toward the monitor on the table when she hears the sound of a baby whimpering. She excuses herself and goes to get Robbie from his nap. After changing his diaper, Bonnie returns with him to the living room.

"Would you like to hold him?" she asks Gloria. Gloria nods, and Bonnie gently places Robbie in her outstretched arms. As the two women coo over the baby, the father trains his video camera on mothers and child.

Notes

CHAPTER 1

1. U.S. Congress, Office of Technology Assessment, *Infertility: Medical and Social Choices*, OTA-BA-358 (Washington, D.C.: Government Printing Office, 1988), p. 35 (hereafter cited as OTA Report).

2. Ibid., p. 6.

3. Adoption provisions based on those in New Jersey as reported in Cecilia Zalkind, "Adoption Law, Policy and Practice in New Jersey" (paper prepared in 1988 for the Task Force on New Reproductive Practices, in conjunction with the New Jersey Bioethics Commission), p. 1.

4. Ibid., pp. 12–13.

5. OTA Report, p. 107.

6. Cited in Richard John Neuhaus, "The Return of Eugenics," *Commentary*, April 1988, p. 16.

7. Ibid.

8. Paul Ramsey, "Shall We 'Reproduce'?" *Journal of the American Medical Association* 220 (June 12, 1972): 1484.

9. Ibid.

10. Ibid.

11. Leon R. Kass, *Toward a More Natural Science: Biology and Human Affairs* (New York: Free Press, 1985), p. 101.

12. Ibid., p. 109.

13. Neuhaus, "The Return of Eugenics," p. 15.

14. OTA Report, p. 36.

15. Ibid., p. 98.

16. Account taken from the testimony of Kathryn Quick, presented orally at a public hearing of the New Jersey Commission on Legal and Ethical Problems in the Delivery of Health Care (New Jersey Bioethics Commission), held in Newark, N.J., (hereafter Bioethics Commission hearing).

17. Ibid.

CHAPTER 2

1. Factual details taken from OTA Report, p. 41.

2. Etienne-Emile Baulieu, "Contragestion and Other Clinical Applications of RU 486, an Antiprogesterone at the Receptor," *Science* 245 (September 1989): 1356.

3. *Smith v. Hartigan*, 556 F.Supp. 157 (N.D. Ill.) (1983), cited in OTA Report, p. 253.

4. OTA Report, p. 253.

5. Rebecca J. Cook, "Antiprogestin Drugs: Medical and Legal Issues," *Family Planning Perspectives* 21 (1989): 267.

6. Ibid.

7. Congregation for the Doctrine of the Faith, *Instruction on Respect for Human Life in Its Origin and on the Dignity of Procreation* (Vatican City, 1987); Sacred Congregation for the Doctrine of the Faith, *Declaration on Procured Abortion* (1974), cited in OTA Report, p. 208.

8. Cook, "Antiprogestin Drugs," p. 267.

9. OTA Report, p. 128.

10. Ibid., p. 41.

11. Ibid., pp. 117, 128.

12. Ibid., p. 128.

13. Rev. Robert Harahan, "Keynote Address—Natural Family Planning Convention at Seton Hall, June, 1987," *Linacre Quarterly*, May 1988, p. 42.

14. Ibid., p. 45 (original emphasis).

15. Ibid., pp. 47, 49.

16. Ibid., p. 46.

17. OTA Report, p. 365.

18. Ibid., pp. 123–24.

19. Harahan, "Keynote Address," p. 48.

20. Susan Sherwin, *No Longer Patient: Feminist Ethics and Health Care* (Philadelphia: Temple University Press, 1992), p. 129.

21. Ibid., pp. 84, 127.

22. Ibid., esp. chaps. 4 and 6.

23. Ibid.

24. Ibid., p. 61.

25. Ibid., p. 63.

26. LeRoy Walters, "Ethics and New Reproductive Technologies: An International Review of Committee Statements," *Hastings Center Report* 17, spec. supp. (June 1987): p. 4.

27. George J. Annas, "Redefining Parenthood and Protecting Embryos: Why We Need New Laws," *Hastings Center Report* 14 (October 1984): 50.

28. John A. Robertson, "In the Beginning: The Legal Status of Early Embryos," *Virginia Law Review* 76 (April 1990): 459.

29. The account of the Davis case is taken from George J. Annas, "A French Homunculus in a Tennessee Court," *Hastings Center Report* 19 (1989): 20–22.

30. John A. Robertson, "Resolving Disputes over Frozen Embryos," *Hastings Center Report* 19 (November–December 1989): 7.

31. Ibid., p. 8.

32. "New Turn in a Couple's Fight over Embryos," *New York Times*, May 27, 1990.

33. *Davis v. Davis*, 1990 Tenn. App. LEXIS 642 (Tenn. Ct. App. September 13, 1990).

34. *Davis v. Davis*, 842 S.N. 2d 588, 1992 Tenn. LEXIS 400 (Tenn. 1992).

35. Robertson, "Resolving Disputes," p. 9.

36. Ibid., p. 11.

37. "Medical Technology and the Law," *Harvard Law Review* 103 (May 1990): 1544.

38. Robertson, "In the Beginning," p. 503.

39. This account is based on an April 1993 segment of *Sally Jessy Raphael*, on which I appeared as a guest.

40. "7 Embryos in Custody Case Are Destroyed," *New York Times*, June 16, 1993, p. A18.

41. Harahan, "Keynote Address," p. 44.

CHAPTER 3

1. Charles Krauthammer, "The Ethics of Human Manufacture," *New Republic*, May 4, 1987, pp. 17–21.

2. Ibid., p. 18.

3. Ibid., p. 20.

4. Ibid., p. 21.

5. OTA Report, p. 285.

6. Larry Gostin, ed., *Surrogate Motherhood: Politics and Privacy* (Bloomington: Indiana University Press, 1990), App. II, p. 261.

7. New Jersey Commission on Legal and Ethical Problems in the Delivery of Health Care, *After Baby M: The Legal, Ethical, and Social Dimensions of Surrogacy* (n.p., September 1992), p. 91 n. 28 (hereafter New Jersey Bioethics Commission, *After Baby M*).

8. The features described are based on provisions of New York State Senate Bill 1429-A (Dunne-Goodhue bill), introduced during the 1987–88 session.

9. In ibid., para. 119.

10. Ibid., para. 122 (b).

11. Ibid., para. 122 (g), (j).

12. This description is based on provisions of the surrogacy law passed in Florida: FLA. STAT. sec. 63.212(1) (1988).

13. The features of the law described here are essentially those of the law passed in Michigan: MICH. COMP. LAWS sec. 722.851 (1988).

14. Ibid.

15. Larry Gostin, "A Civil Liberties Analysis of Surrogacy Arrangements," *Law, Medicine, and Health Care* 16 (1988): 7. Many of the points articulated in this discussion are drawn from the Gostin article. See also John Robertson, "Surrogate Mothers: Not So Novel After All," *Hastings Center Report* 13 (October 1983): 28–34.

16. Gostin, "Civil Liberties Analysis," p. 8.

17. Ibid., citing *Santosky v. Kramer*, 455 U.S. 745, 753 (1982).

18. Gostin, "Civil Liberties Analysis," p. 8.

19. The views presented next are taken from testimony offered by Gary Skoloff

(attorney for William Stern in the Baby M case) at Bioethics Commission hearing.

20. Gostin, "Civil Liberties Analysis," p. 10.

21. George J. Annas, "Protecting the Liberty of Pregnant Patients," *New England Journal of Medicine* 316 (May 7, 1987): 1213.

22. ARK. STAT. ANN. sec. 9-10-201(b) (1989).

23. Noel Keane, "Legal Problems of Surrogate Motherhood," *Southern Illinois University Law Journal* 47 (1980): 439.

24. This account is taken from "Statement of New Jersey Catholic Conference in Connection with Public Hearing on Surrogate Mothering," signed by William F. Bolan, Jr., Executive Director of the New Jersey Catholic Conference (document submitted as part of Bioethics Commission hearing). Portions of the text are quoted verbatim in the presentation attributed here to Father Reardon.

25. Cited in Lori B. Andrews, "Surrogate Motherhood: The Challenge for Feminists," *Law, Medicine, and Health Care* 16 (1988): 72.

26. Joan Mahoney, "An Essay on Surrogacy and Feminist Thought," *Law, Medicine, and Health Care* 16 (1988): 81.

27. Testimony of Gena Corea, associate director of the Institute on Women and Technology, before California Assembly Judiciary Committee, April 5, 1988; reprinted as "Junk Liberty" in Gostin, *Surrogate Motherhood*, pp. 325–37 (quotation, p. 325).

28. Ibid., pp. 325–26.

29. Ibid., p. 333.

30. This account is taken from Ruth Macklin, "Is There Anything Wrong with Surrogate Motherhood? An Ethical Analysis," *Law, Medicine, and Health Care* 16 (1988): 57–64; reprinted in Gostin, *Surrogate Motherhood*, pp. 136–50.

31. Hallye Jordan, "Surrogate Parenting Sanctions Suggested," *Los Angeles Daily Journal*, July 18, 1990, p. 5.

32. Sidney Callahan, "No Child Wants to Live in a Womb for Hire," *National Catholic Reporter*, October 11, 1985.

33. Sidney Callahan, quoted in Iver Peterson, "Baby M Trial Splits Ranks of Feminists," *New York Times*, February 24, 1987, p. B1.

34. *Commonwealth of Kentucky v. Surrogate Parenting Associates, Inc.* (October 26, 1983), Kentucky Circuit Court, Franklin County.

35. The arguments in this section are excerpted from Ruth Macklin, " 'Due' and 'Undue' Inducements: On Paying Money to Research Subjects," *IRB: A Review of Human Subjects Research* 3 (May 1981): 1–6.

36. Mahoney, "Essay on Surrogacy," p. 81.

37. See Leon R. Kass, " 'Making Babies' Revisited," *Public Interest* 54 (Winter 1979): 32–60.

38. National Organ Transplant Act of 1984, 42 U.S.C. 274(e) (1982).

39. See Margaret Jane Radin, "Market-Inalienability," *Harvard Law Review* 100 (June 1987): 1849–1937.

40. Bolan, "Statement of New Jersey Catholic Conference," p. 5.

41. OTA report, pp. 261, 285, 287, 288.

CHAPTER 4

1. L. M. Purdy, "Genetic Diseases: Can Having Children Be Immoral?" in *Moral Problems in Medicine*, ed. Samuel Gorovitz et al., 2d ed. (Englewood Cliffs, N.J.: Prentice-Hall, 1983), p. 377.

2. More than half the agencies that provide matching services require some sort of psychological screening or counseling; however, a survey carried out by the Office of Technology Assessment (OTA Report, p. 270) does not make clear the extent of that counseling.

3. OTA Report, p. 272. See also W. R. Frederick, R. Delaphenha, G. Gray, et al., "HIV Testing on Surrogate Mothers," *New England Journal of Medicine* 317 (1987): 1351–52.

4. A provision of one of two bills proposed in New Jersey. See Lori Andrews, "The Aftermath of Baby M: Proposed State Laws on Surrogate Motherhood," *Hastings Center Report* 17 (October–November 1987): 35.

5. Figures for these procedures reported in an OTA survey conducted in 1986 and contained in OTA Report, p. 141, supply a median cost of $4,688 for IVF with embryo replacement in the same woman; the higher figure represents the added medical costs of treating an additional patient.

6. OTA Report, p. 273.

7. Paul J. Fink, foreword to *Premenstrual Syndrome: Ethical and Legal Implications in a Biomedical Perspective*, ed. B. E. Ginsburg and B. F. Carter (New York: Plenum Press, 1987), pp. x–xi.

8. Ibid., p. ix.

9. Provisions of the agreement set forth here are based on the surrogacy parenting agreement between William Stern and Mary Beth Whitehead, disputants in the Baby M case (hereafter, Stern-Whitehead surrogacy agreement). Copies of the agreement were distributed to members of the New Jersey Bioethics Commission's Task Force on New Reproductive Practices, of which the author was a member.

10. The blood test to diagnose pregnancy is normally obtained eleven to fourteen days after embryo replacement.

11. Excerpt based on Stern-Whitehead surrogacy agreement.

CHAPTER 5

1. John C. Fletcher, "Ethical Issues in Genetic Screening, Prenatal Diagnosis, and Counseling," in *Ethical Issues at the Outset of Life*, ed. William B. Weil, Jr., and Martin Benjamin (Boston: Blackwell Scientific Publications, 1987), p. 77.

2. Michael Craft, "The Current Status of XYY and XXY Syndromes: A Review of Treatment Implications," in *Biology, Crime, and Ethics*, ed. Frank H. Marsh and Janet Katz (Cincinnati, Ohio: Anderson, 1985), p. 114.

3. Fletcher, "Ethical Issues," p. 77.

4. Craft, "Current Status," p. 114.

5. Ibid., pp. 114–15.

6. Margaret O'Brien Steinfels and Carol Levine, eds., "The XYY Controversy: Researching Violence and Genetics," *Hastings Center Report* 10, spec. supp. (August 1980): 16.

7. Ibid., p. 17. See also Craft, "Current Status," p. 115.

8. Craft, "Current Status," p. 117.

9. Ibid., p. 118.

10. Steinfels and Levine, "The XYY Controversy," p. 22.

11. Ibid.

12. George J. Annas, "Baby M: Babies (and Justice) for Sale," *Hastings Center Report* 17 (June 1987): 15.

13. Based on para. 13 of Stern-Whitehead surrogacy agreement.

14. Ibid.

15. Craft, "Current Status," p. 115.

16. Susan E. Bell, "Premenstrual Syndrome and the Medicalization of Menopause: A Sociological Perspective," in *Premenstrual Syndrome: Ethical and Legal Implications in a Biomedical Perspective*, ed. B. E. Ginsburg and B. F. Carter (New York: Plenum Press, 1987), p. 153.

17. Material in this section on MBD is extracted from Ruth Macklin, "Therapy and Social Control," chap. 4 in *Man, Mind, and Morality: The Ethics of Behavior Control* (Englewood Cliffs, N.J.: Prentice-Hall, 1982), pp. 66–67.

18. This material on XYY and genetic determinism is taken from Ruth Macklin, "The Premenstrual Syndrome (PMS) Label: Benefit or Burden?" in Ginsburg and Carter, *Premenstrual Syndrome*, p. 23.

19. Willard Gaylin, Ruth Macklin, and Tabitha M. Powledge, eds., *Violence and the Politics of Research* (New York: Plenum Press, 1981), pp. 98–119.

20. Material on the medicalization of PMS is taken from Bell, "Premenstrual Syndrome," pp. 155–67.

21. Ibid., p. 155.

22. Ibid., p. 157.

23. Ibid., pp. 164–67.

24. Virginia Cassara, "A View from the Top of a Consumer Organization," in Ginsburg and Carter, *Premenstrual Syndrome*, p. 208. Facts about PMS Action, Inc., and other views expressed in these paragraphs are based on this article (pp. 207–12).

25. Ibid., p. 208.

26. Ibid., p. 209.

27. P.M.S. O'Brien, "Controversies in Premenstrual Syndrome: Etiology and Treatment," in Ginsburg and Carter, *Premenstrual Syndrome*, p. 317.

28. Ibid.

29. Ibid., p. 319.

30. Ibid., p. 324.

31. Ibid.

32. Cassara, "View from the Top," p. 210.

33. Description of cases that follow are taken from Christopher Boorse, "Premenstrual Syndrome and Criminal Responsibility," in Ginsburg and Carter, *Premenstrual Syndrome*, pp. 81–87.

34. Ibid., p. 83.

35. Ibid., pp. 84–85.

36. The account of *People v. Santos* (November 3, 1982, No. 1K046229, Crim. Ct. N.Y.) is taken from Boorse, "Premenstrual Syndrome," p. 85. The real name of the attorney, a Legal Aid lawyer, was Stephanie Benson.

37. Details of this case, which occurred in England, are taken from Katharina Dalton, "Should Premenstrual Syndrome Be a Legal Defense?" in Ginsburg and Carter, *Premenstrual Syndrome*, pp. 288–89.

38. Boorse, "Premenstrual Syndrome," p. 87.

39. Dalton, "Legal Defense," p. 293.

40. Robert L. Sadoff, "The Insanity Defense in Criminal Law," in Ginsburg and Carter, *Premenstrual Syndrome*, p. 74.

41. Ibid., p. 77, citing the Insanity Defense Reform Act of 1984, sec. 20 (a) and (b).

42. Sadoff, "Insanity Defense," pp. 77–78.

43. Cassara, "View from the Top," p. 211.

44. *Time*, July 27, 1981, quoted in Mary Brown Parlee, "Media Treatment of Premenstrual Syndrome," in Ginsburg and Carter, *Premenstrual Syndrome*, p. 190.

45. *Washington Post*, July 10, 1981, quoted in Parlee, "Media Treatment," p. 192.

46. *Harper's Bazaar*, November 1975, quoted in Parlee, "Media Treatment," p. 191.

47. Bell, "Premenstrual Syndrome," p. 167.

48. Ibid. The article cited is R. L. Reid and S.S.C. Yen, "Premenstrual Syndrome," *American Journal of Obstetrics and Gynecology* 139 (1981): 85–104.

49. C. R. Jeffery, "Criminal Law, Biological Psychiatry, and Premenstrual Syndrome: Conflicting Perspectives," in Ginsburg and Carter, *Premenstrual Syndrome*, p. 131.

50. Ibid., pp. 139–40.

51. Ibid.

52. Ibid., p. 142. A PET scan (positron emission tomography) is an advanced form of x-ray.

CHAPTER 6

1. *Vitaly Tarasoff et al. v. The Regents of the University of California et al.*, 551 P.2d 334, 17 Cal. 3d 425, Supreme Court of California, In Bank, July 1, 1976.

2. Ibid.

3. Howard Zonana, Michael Norko, and David Stier, "The AIDS Patient on the Psychiatric Unit: Ethical and Legal Issues," *Psychiatric Annals* 18 (1988): 587–93.

4. Ibid., p. 591.

5. D. C. Harvey and L. U. Trivelli, "HIV Education for Persons with Mental Disabilities," *AIDS Technical Report* (Washington, D.C.: National Association of Protection & Advocacy Systems, 1990), p. 6.

6. Paul S. Appelbaum, "AIDS, Psychiatry, and the Law," *Hospital and Community Psychiatry* 39 (1988): 14.

7. Ibid.

8. Zonana, Norko, and Stier, "The AIDS Patient," pp. 591–92.

CHAPTER 7

1. Based on para. 15 of Stern-Whitehead surrogacy agreement.

2. Martha A. Field, "Controlling the Woman to Protect the Fetus," *Law, Medicine, and Health Care* 17 (1989): 118.

3. Isabel Wilkerson, "Jury in Illinois Refuses to Charge Mother in Drug Death of Newborn," *New York Times*, May 27, 1989, p. 10.

4. *Jennifer Clarise Johnson v. State of Florida*, Case No. 89-1765, Florida Court of Appeals, Fifth District, 1991 Fla. App. LEXIS 3583, filed April 18, 1991.

5. Ibid., LEXIS NEXIS, 1st CASE of Level 1 printed in full format, p. 3.

6. Mark Hansen, "Courts Side with Moms in Drug Cases," *ABA Journal*, November 1992, p. 18.

7. "Pregnant Drug User Taken to Court," *New York Times*, April 27, 1984.

8. Nancy K. Rhoden, "Informed Consent in Obstetrics: Some Special Problems," *Western New England Law Review* 9 (1987): 82.

9. Ibid.

10. Field, "Controlling the Woman," p. 115.

11. George J. Annas, "Baby M: Babies (and Justice) for Sale," *Hastings Center Report* 17 (June 1987): 15.

12. Sherman Elias and George J. Annas, "Social Policy Considerations in Noncoital Reproduction," *Journal of the American Medical Association* 255 (January 3, 1986): 64–65.

13. Details about the California case are taken from William Vogeler, "Unique Surrogacy Lawsuit Seeking Custody, Money," *Los Angeles Daily Journal*, August 14, 1990, p. 1.

14. Ibid.

CHAPTER 8

1. Veronika E. B. Kolder, Janet Gallagher, and Michael T. Parsons, "Court-Ordered Obstetrical Interventions," *New England Journal of Medicine* 316 (May 7, 1987): pp. 1192–96.

2. George J. Annas, "Protecting the Liberty of Pregnant Patients," *New England Journal of Medicine* 316 (May 7, 1987): 1213.

3. Michael C. Copeman, letter to the editor, *New England Journal of Medicine* 317 (November 5, 1987): 1223–24.

4. Michelle Harrison, "The Baby with Two Mothers," op-ed piece in *Wall Street Journal*, October 24, 1990.

CHAPTER 9

1. This draft of a living will for AIDS patients, with the accompanying power-of-attorney document, was developed by Alice Herb, J.D., during her tenure in the Department of Epidemiology and Social Medicine at Montefiore Medical Center, Bronx, N.Y.

2. "Patient Choice: Maternal-Fetal Conflict," ACOG Committee Opinion No. 55, October 1987.

3. From a proposed hospital policy described in Ruth Macklin, "The Inner Workings of an Ethics Committee: Latest Battle over Jehovah's Witnesses," *Hastings Center Report* 18 (February–March 1988): 19.

4. Ibid., p. 20.

5. New York State Task Force on Life and the Law, *Surrogate Parenting: Analysis and Recommendations for Public Policy*, (N.p., May 1988), p. 118.

6. This decision was reached by the New York State Task Force and published in ibid.; also stated in New Jersey Bioethics Commission, *After Baby M.*

7. OTA Report, p. 284; the case cited is *Smith & Smith v. Jones & Jones*, 85-532014DZ, Detroit, Mich., 3d Dist. (March 15, 1986), as reported in *BioLaw*, ed. James Childress, Patricia King, Karen Rothenberg, et al. (Frederick, Md.: University Publishers of America, 1986). See also George J. Annas, "The Baby Broker Boom," *Hastings Center Report* 16 (June 1986): 30–31.

8. The account that follows is adapted from Ruth Macklin, "Artificial Means of Reproduction and Our Understanding of the Family," *Hastings Center Report* 21 (January–February, 1991): 5–11.

9. Sherman Elias and George J. Annas, "Noncoital Reproduction," *Journal of the American Medical Association* 255 (January 3, 1986): p. 67.

10. George J. Annas, "Death without Dignity for Commercial Surrogacy: The Case of Baby M," *Hastings Center Report* 18 (April–May 1988): 23.

11. Quoted in Annas, "The Baby Broker Boom," p. 31.

12. Sidney Callahan, "The Ethical Challenge of the New Reproductive Technology," paper presented to the Task Force on New Reproductive Practices; published in *Medical Ethics: A Guide for Health Care Professionals*, ed. John F. Monagle and David C. Thomasma (Frederick, Md.: Aspen, 1987).

CHAPTER 10

1. *In re*: A.C., Appellant, Court of Appeals, No. 87-609, On Hearing en Banc, p. 1108, n. 2.

2. Appendix A to "Settlement Agreement, Policy on Decision-making by Pregnant Patients at the George Washington University Hospital," p. 1. The medical center's policy is based on the settlement agreement, November 21, 1990, between Nettie Stoner and Daniel Stoner and George Washington University Medical Center. The civil rights and medical malpractice suit, *Stoners v. G.W.U.*, which culminated in this agreement, was brought by the ACLU Reproductive Freedom Project on behalf of the Stoners, Angela Carder's parents.

3. Ibid., pp. 3, 5.

4. Ibid., pp. 6, 7–8.

5. Ibid., pp. 9, 11.

6. E.g., two New York cases—*In the Matter of Baby Girl L.J.*, 132 Misc. 2d. 972, 505 N.Y.S. 2d. 813 (Surr. Ct. 1986); and *In the Matter of the Adoption of Paul*, 146 Misc. 2d 379, 550 N.Y.S. 2d 815 (Fam. Ct. 1990)—and a Kentucky case, *Surrogate Parenting Associates, Inc. v. Kentucky*, 704 S.W. 2d 209 (Ky. Sup. Ct. 1986).

7. Nos. X-633190 and AD-576, slip op. (Cal. App. Dep't. Super. Ct. Oct 22, 1990), *aff'd*, 234 Cal. App. 3d 1557, 286 Cal. Rptr. 369 (Cal. Ct. App. 1991), *review petition granted*, 4 Cal. Rptr. 2d 170, 822 P. 2d 1317 (Cal. Sup. Ct. 1992).

8. 234 Cal. App. 3d 1557, 1569, 1571–72, 286 Cal. Rptr. 369, 377–78, 379 (Cal. Ct. App. 1991), *review petition granted*, 4 Cal. Rptr. 2d 170, 822 P.2d 1317 (Cal. Sup. Ct. 1992).

9. This was true as of May 31, 1993.

10. Dr. Marshall Klaus, quoted in William Vogeler, "Surrogate Mother's Testimony Details Emotional Attachment," *Los Angeles Daily Journal*, October 11, 1990, p. 2.

11. The statements in this paragraph are based on New Jersey Bioethics Commission, *After Baby M*, pp. 162–67.

12. R. Alta Charo, "Legislative Approaches to Surrogate Motherhood," *Law, Medicine, and Health Care* 16 (1988): 104.

13. Michelle Harrison, "The Baby with Two Mothers," *Wall Street Journal*, October 24, 1990.

14. Remarks based on ibid.

15. Ronald Sullivan, "Judge Lets Gay Partner Adopt Child," *New York Times*, January 31, 1992, p. B1.

16. Carol Levine, "AIDS and Changing Concepts of Family," *Milbank Quarterly* 68, supp. 1 (1990): 36.

17. New Jersey Bioethics Commission, *After Baby M*, p. 154.

18. Philip Carrizosa, "First Appeal of Surrogacy Case Argued," *Los Angeles Daily Journal*, October 20, 1991, pp. 1, 5.

19. New Jersey Bioethics Commission, *After Baby M*, p. 170.

20. Ibid., p. 171.

21. Ibid.

22. Robert E. Gould, "And What About Baby M's Ruined Life?" op-ed piece in *New York Times*, March 26, 1987.

Credits

Portions of this book are reprinted from Ruth Macklin, "The New Sexual Issues: Public Policy Implications," in *Ethical Practice in Psychiatry and the Law, Volume VII of Critical Issues in American Psychiatry and the Law*, ed. Richard Rosner and Robert Weinstock (New York: Plenum Press, 1990), pp. 243–55.

Portions of Chapter 3 are reprinted from Ruth Macklin, "Is There Anything Wrong with Surrogate Motherhood? An Ethical Analysis," *Law, Medicine, and Health Care* 16 (1988): 57–64; and from Ruth Macklin, "'Due' and 'Undue' Inducements: On Paying Money to Research Subjects," *IRB: A Review of Human Subjects Research* 3 (May 1981): 1–6.

Portions of Chapter 5 are reprinted from Ruth Macklin, "Therapy and Social Control," *Man, Mind, and Morality: The Ethics of Behavior Control* (Englewood Cliffs, N.J.: Prentice-Hall, 1982), pp. 66–67; and from Ruth Macklin, "The Premenstrual Syndrome (PMS) Label: Benefit or Burden?" in *Premenstrual Syndrome: Ethical and Legal Implications in a Biomedical Perspective*, ed. B. E. Ginsburg and B. F. Carter (New York: Plenum Press, 1987), pp. 17–30.

Portions of Chapter 9 are reprinted from Ruth Macklin, "The Inner Workings of an Ethics Committee: Latest Battle over Jehovah's Witnesses," *Hastings Center Report* 18 (February–March 1988): 15–20; and from Ruth Macklin, "Artificial Means of Reproduction and Our Understanding of the Family," *Hastings Center Report* 21 (January–February 1991): 5–11. Reproduced by permission. © The Hastings Center.

Portions of Chapter 10 are reprinted from *Enemies of Patients* by Ruth Macklin. Copyright © 1993 by Ruth Macklin. Reprinted by permission of Oxford University Press, Inc.

Index

Criminalization: of artificial reproduction, 41; of commercial surrogacy, 51, 53–54; of noncompliance, 219
Cryopreservation, 31–32, 40, 44; agreement for, 91; risks and benefits of, 91–92
C-section, 158, 173–74, 186–89, 219

Daily Law Journal, 166
Dalton, Katharina, 110, 112, 113, 114, 117, 120
Danger to public health, 143
Davis, Junior L., 42, 43
Davis, Mary Sue, 42, 43, 45
Davis v. Davis, 42–44
Decisional capacity, 181–82
Dehumanization of babies, 59
Diminished capacity plea, 116
Diminished responsibility plea, 114, 116
Directive counseling, 73, 75–77, 79
Disclosure: to insurance companies, 170–71, 177, 178; state law regarding HIV, 130, 139; to psychiatric patients, of exposure to AIDS, 135, 144–45
Disposition of preembryos, 92
Distributive justice, 66, 67
District of Columbia Court of Appeals, on Carder case, 220–21
Draconian procedures, 136–37
Drug trafficking law, 157
Durable Power of Attorney for Health Care Decisions, draft of, 198–99
Duties and obligations: ethical categories of, 140; of surrogate mother during pregnancy, 66
Duty to warn, 125–26, 138–39

Egg donation programs, 15, 80, 179; compared to surrogacy, 225–27
Embryo research, 44–47
Embryos, as property, 44
English, Christine, 113–14

Ethical analysis: of ACOG opinion on patient autonomy, 219; of assisted reproduction, 17–19, 20–24, 38–39; of directive counseling, 72–80; of forced C-section, 188–89; of informed consent versus confidentiality, 141, 183–84; of involuntary commitment, 143; of surrogacy, 61–69, 207–9; of surrogate's claims on child, 210–15, 231–32
"Ethics of Human Manufacture, The," in *New Republic*, 50
Eugenics, 19
Extra Y chromosome, 97–98, 102; and abortion, 99–100, 103; controversy, 98–99; frequency of, 103–4; and medical labeling, 108–9

Family, changing definitions of, 227–29
Family secrets, 226–27
Fate of embryos, 23, 31–32, 34, 40, 50
Fatherhood, 213
Feminist International Network of Resistance to Reproductive and Genetic Engineering (FINRRAGE), 36
Feminist position. *See under* New reproductive technologies; PMS; Surrogacy
Feminists for Life, 60
Fertility drugs. *See* Clomiphene citrate
Fertilization and early development of embryo, 28–31
Fetal alcohol syndrome, 155, 165
Fetal neglect, 167–68
"Fetal police," 29
Fetus, as defined by federal regulations, 45
Florida Supreme Court, on drug trafficking law, 157
Frozen embryos, fate of, 22–23, 40, 42, 44, 92

Genetic determinism, 108–9

Maternal-infant bonding in utero, 224–25
Medicalization of behavior, 106–7, 108–11
Medical labels, 108
Menning, Barbara, 25
Michigan statute on commercial surrogacy, 53–54
M'Naghten test of insanity, 115–16
Models of custody arrangements, 230
Monson case, 156
Mother's right to privacy, 156
Multiple gestation, 33

National Ethics Committee, France, 40
Natural Law, 17–19
New Jersey Supreme Court, on Baby M case, 55, 58, 223
New reproductive technologies: liberal feminist position on, 38–39; radical feminist position on, 36–37, 59–61; Roman Catholic position on, 33–35, 39, 46, 58–59, 70
New York Surrogate Court judge, on adoption by lesbian, 228
NIH (National Institutes of Health), 41
Noncommercial surrogacy, 64, 69, 206–10. *See also* Commercial surrogacy; Surrogacy
NOW, New Jersey chapter, on Baby M case, 60

OTA (Office of Technology Assessment), 241 nn. 2, 5
"Ought implies can" maxim, 76
Ownership of genes, 213

Parent-child bond, 58
Paternalistic arguments, 67, 77, 188
Patient-physician relationship, 95, 203, 221
Patient Self-determination Act, 199
People v. Santos, 114–15

Periluteal phase dysphoric disorder, 88–89, 177. *See also* PMS
Persuasive definition, 66
Physicians' obligation: to preserve confidentiality, 130, 171, 182; to protect psychiatric patients, 127, 130, 136–37, 143–44; to provide complete information, 145, 171; to treat, 182
PMS, 105; diagnosis of, 88–89; dietary recommendations for, 121; eclectic treatment of, 176–77; etiology of, 111; as legal defense, 113–16, 120; and medical labeling, 117–20; medicalization of, 106, 109–11; placebo effect and, 111–12; PMS Action, 110–11; progesterone for, 109–11, 113, 115; screening for, 118–19; women's movement and, 117–20
Pneumocystis carinii pneumonia, 171
Postbirth sanctions, 156
Posttraumatic stress syndrome, 12
Preembryo, 30–31, 40–44
Pregnancy: court-ordered intervention during, 159–60; medical definition of, 29–30; reduction, 33
Pregnant women: coercion of, 158–59, 188–89, 201–2; and fetal conflict, 188, 200–202, 219; respect for autonomy of, 200, 219, 221; rights of, 156–57, 186, 188–89, 201–2; substance abuse and, 156–57
Prenatal screening, 37–38
Preventive detention, 140–41
Procreative autonomy, 44
Procreative freedom, 55–57
Procreative liberty, 61, 227
Progesterone. *See under* PMS
Psychiatric evaluation of surrogate, 51, 101, 166
Psychiatric patients: and confidentiality, 126–27, 178; informed consent and, 131; involuntary commitment of, 143; rights of, 131, 137, 143–44;